Spreading Improvement Across Your Health Care Organization

Edited by Kevin M. Nolan, M.A., and Marie W. Schall, M.A.

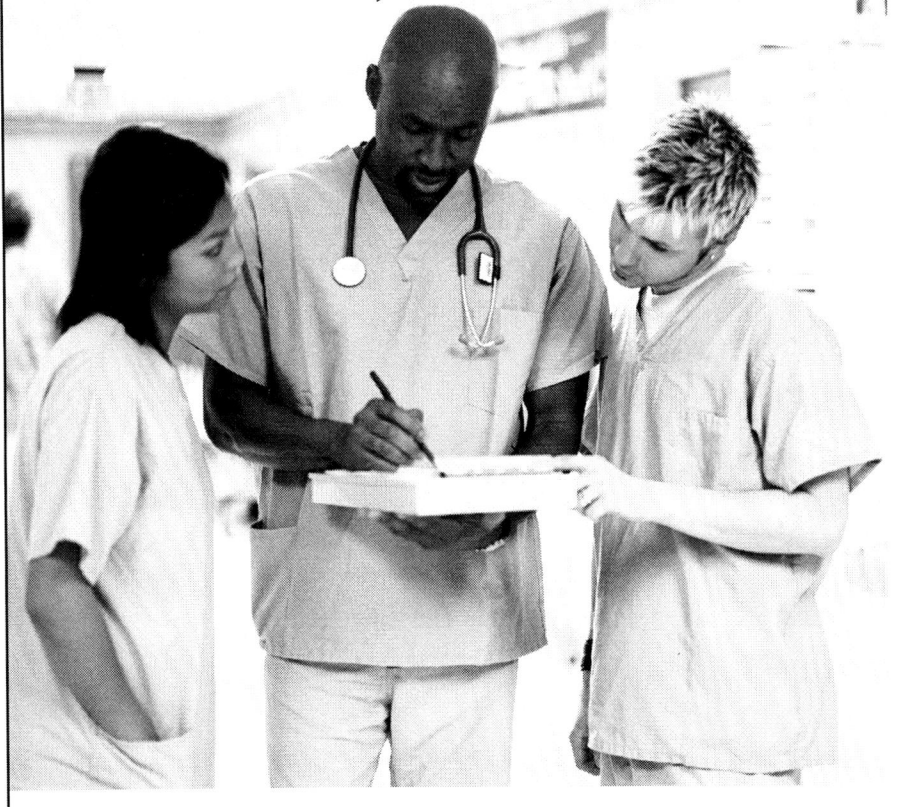

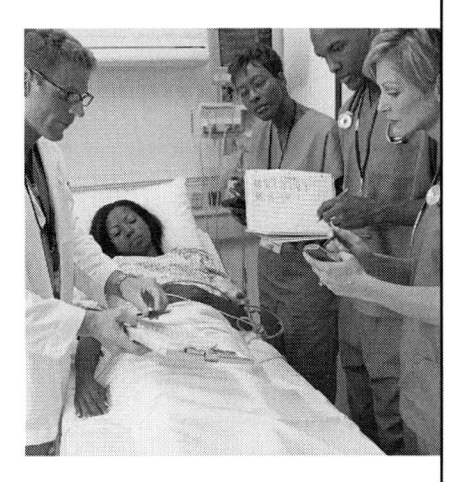

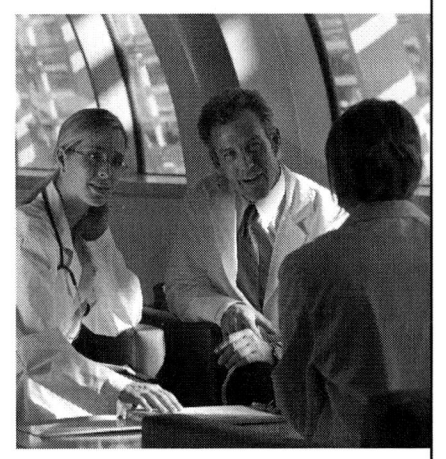

Joint Commission Resources

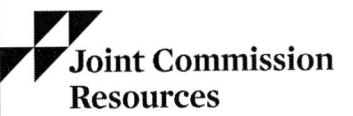

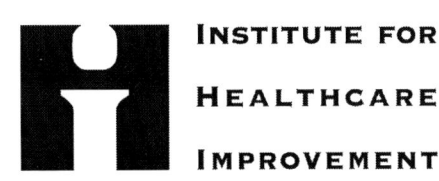

INSTITUTE FOR HEALTHCARE IMPROVEMENT

Executive Editor: Steven Berman
Project Manager: Christine Wyllie
Editorial Coordinator: Noel C. Wagner
Associate Director, Production: Johanna Harris
Executive Director: Catherine Chopp Hinckley, Ph.D.
Vice President, Learning: Charles Macfarlane, F.A.C.H.E.
Joint Commission/JCR Reviewers: David Boan, Eileen Chabot, Robin Little, Louise Kuhny, Deborah Nadzam

Joint Commission Resources Mission
The mission of Joint Commission Resources is to continuously improve the safety and quality of care in the United States and in the international community through the provision of education and consultation services and international accreditation.

Joint Commission Resources educational programs and publications support, but are separate from, the accreditation activities of The Joint Commission. Attendees at Joint Commission Resources educational programs and purchasers of Joint Commission Resources publications receive no special consideration or treatment in, or confidential information about, the accreditation process.

The inclusion of an organization name, product, or service in a Joint Commission publication should not be construed as an endorsement of such organization, product, or services, nor is failure to include an organization name, product, or service to be construed as disapproval.

© 2007 by Joint Commission on Accreditation of Healthcare Organizations and the Institute for Healthcare Improvement

Joint Commission Resources, Inc. (JCR), a not-for-profit affiliate of The Joint Commission, has been designated by the Joint Commission to publish publications and multimedia products. JCR reproduces and distributes these materials under license from the Joint Commission.

The Institute for Healthcare Improvement (IHI) is a not-for-profit organization helping to lead the improvement of health care throughout the world. Founded in 1991 and based in Cambridge, Massachusetts, IHI works to accelerate change by cultivating promising concepts for improving patient care and turning those ideas into action.

All rights reserved. No part of this publication may be reproduced in any form or by any means without written permission from the publisher.

Printed in the U.S.A. 5 4 3 2 1

Requests for permission to make copies of any part of this work should be sent to
Permissions Editor
Department of Publications
Joint Commission Resources
One Renaissance Boulevard
Oakbrook Terrace, Illinois 60181
permissions@jcrinc.com

ISBN: 978-1-59940-106-5
Library of Congress Control Number: 2007932134
For more information about Joint Commission Resources, please visit http://www.jcrinc.com.

Table of Contents

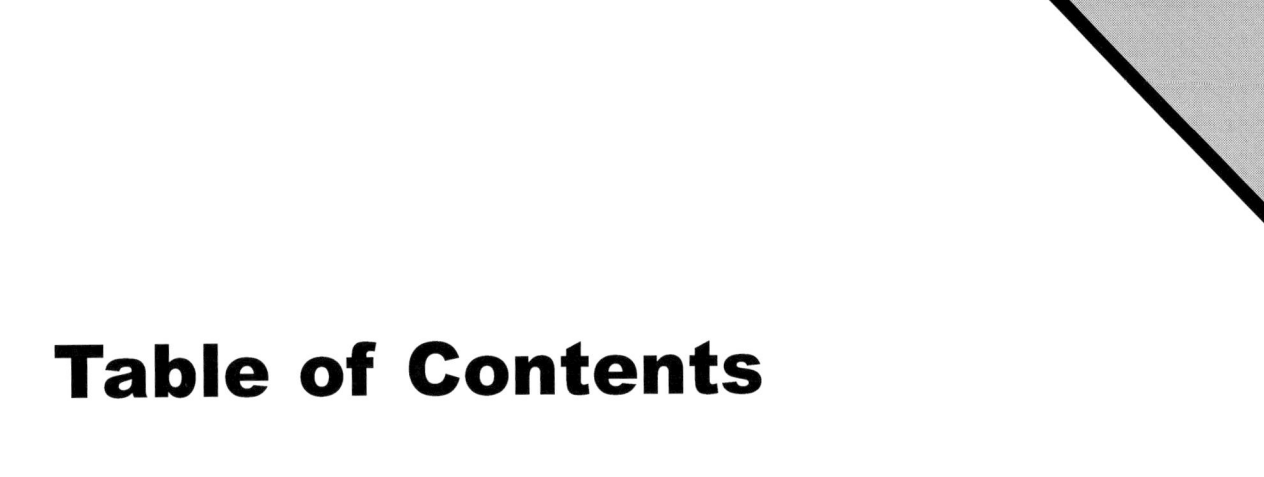

Contributors   v

Foreword   vii
Sir John Oldham, M.B., Ch.B., M.B.A.

Introduction   xi
Kevin M. Nolan, M.A., Marie W. Schall, M.A.

Chapter 1. A Framework for Spread   1
Kevin M. Nolan, M.A., Marie W. Schall, M.A.

Chapter 2. Eliminating Facility-Acquired Pressure Ulcers at Ascension Health   25
Wanda Gibbons, R.N., M.H.A., Helana T. Shanks, R.N.,
Pam Kleinhelter, R.N., M.S.N., Polly Jones, L.C.S.W.

Chapter 3. Preventing Central Line–Associated Bloodstream Infections at Beth Israel Medical Center   41
Brian Koll, M.D., Ina Jabara, R.N., Kathy Peterson, R.N.,
David Crimmins, R.N., C.I.C., Alexis Raimondi, R.N., C.I.C.,
Samuel Acquah, M.D., Hosam Sayed, M.D.

Chapter 4. Spreading the Nurse Knowledge Exchange Handoff Practices at Kaiser Permanente   55
Lisa Schilling, R.N., M.P.H., Chris McCarthy, M.B.A., M.P.H.

Chapter 5. Redesigning Chronic Illness Care in a Public Hospital System   77
Karen Scott Collins, M.D., M.P.H., Reba Williams, M.D.

Chapter 6. Improving Dialysis Care: A Successful National Spread Initiative   95
Carol Beasley, M.P.P.M., Vickie J. Peters, M.S.N., M.A.E.D., R.N., C.P.H.Q., Lawrence Spergel, M.D.

Chapter 7. Insights and Conclusions   113
Kevin M. Nolan, M.A., Marie W. Schall, M.A.

Index   121

Contributors

JCR gratefully acknowledges the contributions of the Institute for Healthcare Improvement (IHI).

Kevin M. Nolan, M.A.
Partner, Associates in Process Improvement,
Silver Spring, Maryland
Senior Fellow, Institute for Healthcare Improvement,
Cambridge, Massachusetts

Marie W. Schall, M.A.
Director, Institute for Healthcare Improvement,
Cambridge, Massachusetts

Foreword

Sir John Oldham, M.B., Ch.B., M.B.A.
General Practitioner, Glossop, United Kingdom
Founder and former Head of the National Primary Care Development Team, Manchester, United Kingdom

Chapter 2. Eliminating Facility-Acquired Pressure Ulcers at Ascension Health

Wanda Gibbons, R.N., M.H.A.
Vice President, Patient Care Services and Chief Nursing Officer, St. Vincent's Medical Center, Jacksonville, Florida

Helana T. Shanks, R.N.
Clinical Resource Coordinator, St. Vincent's Medical Center, Jacksonville, Florida

Pam Kleinhelter, R.N., M.S.N.
Nurse Manager, Intensive Care Unit, St. Vincent's Medical Center, Jacksonville, Florida

Polly Jones, L.C.S.W., C.P.U.Q.
Director, Clinical Excellence, Ascension Health, St. Louis

Chapter 3. Preventing Central Line–Associated Bloodstream Infections at Beth Israel Medical Center

Brian Koll, M.D.
Attending, Department of Medicine, and Chief, Infection Control, Hospital Epidemiologist, Beth Israel Medical Center, New York City, and Associate Professor of Clinical Medicine, Albert Einstein College of Medicine, Bronx, New York

Ina Jabara, R.N.
Nurse Manager, Medical Intensive Care Unit, Beth Israel Medical Center, New York City

Kathy Peterson, R.N.
Nurse Manager, Intensive Care Unit, Beth Israel Medical Center, Kings Highway Division, Brooklyn, New York

David Crimmins, R.N., C.I.C.
Infection Control Practitioner, Beth Israel Medical Center, New York City

Alexis Raimondi, R.N., C.I.C.
Infection Control Manager, Beth Israel Medical Center, New York City

Samuel Acquah, M.D.
Attending, Department of Medicine, Division of Pulmonary Medicine and Critical Care, Beth Israel Medical Center, New York City

Hosam Sayed, M.D.
Attending, Department of Medicine, Division of Pulmonary Medicine and Critical Care, Beth Israel Medical Center, Kings Highway Division, Brooklyn, New York

Chapter 4. Spreading the Nurse Knowledge Exchange Handoff Practices at Kaiser Permanente

Lisa Schilling, R.N., M.P.H.
Director, Healthcare Performance Improvement and Execution Strategy, Kaiser Permanente, Oakland, California

Chris McCarthy, M.B.A., M.P.H.
Director, Innovation Learning Network, Kaiser Permanente, Oakland, California

Chapter 5. Redesigning Chronic Illness Care in a Public Hospital System

Karen Scott Collins, M.D., M.P.H.
Deputy Chief Medical Officer, Health Care Quality and Clinical Services, New York City Health and Hospitals Corporation, New York City

Reba Williams, M.D.
Senior Director, Healthcare Quality Improvement and Innovation, New York City Health and Hospitals Corporation, New York City

Chapter 6. Improving Dialysis Care: A Successful National Spread Initiative

Carol Beasley, M.P.P.M.
Director of Strategic Projects, Institute for Healthcare Improvement, Cambridge, Massachusetts

Vickie J. Peters, M.S.N., M.A.E.D., R.N., C.P.H.Q.
National Coordinator, Fistula First Breakthrough Initiative, Southern California Renal Disease Council, Inc., Los Angeles

Lawrence Spergel, M.D.
Clinical Chair, Fistula First Breakthrough Initiative, San Francisco

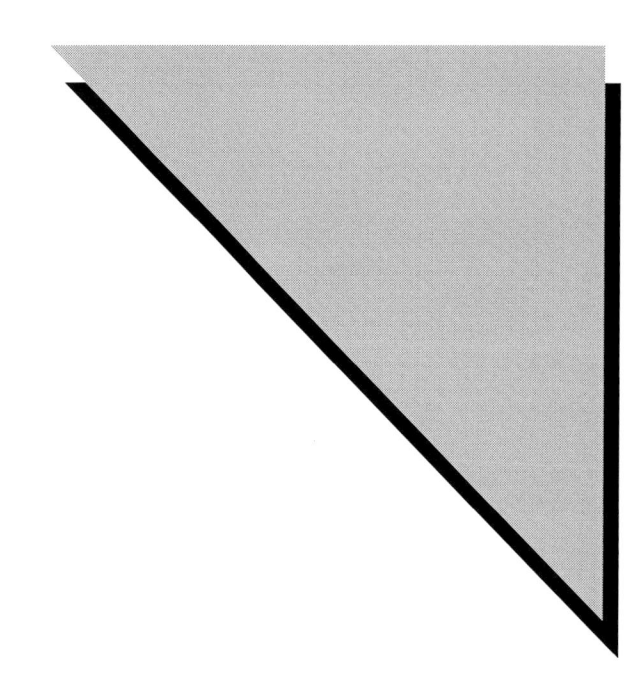

Foreword

Sir John Oldham, M.B., Ch.B., M.B.A.

In January 2000, I was sitting in a hotel in Tampa, Florida, explaining to Tom Nolan and Don Berwick what I had been charged to do by the then-Minister of Health in the United Kingdom, John Denham. The Blair government was focusing on improving the quality of health care in the National Health Service (NHS). I had had conversations about using collaboratives and improvement science to achieve substantial gains in quality improvement, with the result that I was now being asked to use these methods to improve two areas of concern in primary care: (1) access (it was not unusual to have to wait three weeks for a routine appointment with a provider) and (2) the management of coronary heart disease (CHD). The Rogers curve of diffusion of innovation[1] and the "tipping point" of 20% of the population[2] were well understood by the Department of Health, and I was asked that the targets for improvement in access (everyone seen routinely within 48 hours) and CHD (in a variety of parameters, including reduction in mortality) be achieved by 20% of the population of England within two years. At the end of 1999, I had sat with a blank piece of paper and begun to sketch out how I might achieve that, including recruiting and training a core set of people within three months to form a new team—the National Primary Care Development Team.

Three things were clear to me at that stage. First, we needed to plan for spread from the outset and that the concept of conducting pilot tests and evaluating them before rolling out across the NHS was not an option. Continuous evaluation and adjustment needed to be built in. Second, we were not going to do it on our own—rather, we would need to create an infrastructure as we progressed and, more crucially, we would need capacity and capability in the system, a guerrilla army of clinicians who would facilitate and assist with the spread on the basis of their own experience. Finally, the social and psychological aspects of change were going to be as crucial as the methodology. I outlined the task to Tom and Don and presented my embryonic plan. I can picture now in my mind's eye the mixture of anxiety and sympathy that filled their expressions. After a contemplative pause, Tom said, with all the encouragement he could muster, "Well, John, if you achieve this, you will be breaking new frontiers in improvement science and spread."

Thus began a friendship and an exchange of ideas, as well as many years' joint experience and resulting knowledge about how to spread better ideas and practices. This accumulated knowledge is expertly outlined in the Framework for Spread, as presented by Kevin Nolan and Marie Schall in Chapter 1, and brilliantly applied by the authors of the case studies, who tailor the components and sequence of the framework to their own organizations. For the framework is not intended to be a set of rules. That said, it will become obvious to the reader of Chapters 2 through 6 that there are commonalities that cannot be escaped. The topic for spread has to be key and strategic to the organization, with strong and visible leadership presence. There has to be a good evidence base for the topic, and gaining early examples is crucial. Organizational incentives and policies have to be aligned. Communication is crucial; in particular, communicating early sustained gains to the whole organization is very powerful in recruiting the next teams for spread—it gets them thinking in advance. I would go further by saying that when you are contemplating spread on a massive scale, then what you are undertaking is a mixture of marketing and campaigning, with messages segmented to different cohorts of your target audience.

So how did we do in our own task in England? We set about covering 20% of the population by operating four national waves of a collaborative, with monthly data being supplied by all participating practices. The examples created from one wave were used to populate presentations for another wave, with the clinicians and project leads taught in more depth about improvement science as we went along. Adjustments were made in light of continuous evaluation. At one stage, we were running learning workshops for different waves every four weeks. We achieved the coverage in the time set with results that achieved the goals of the collaborative (including 48-hour access for routine matters). However, we went further. The success created the demand for more—both from leaders of the NHS and also other practices who wished to participate, having heard of the scheme from colleagues or from articles we placed in various professional newspapers. We created a national infrastructure of 10 regional centers from sites on the early waves who bid to become centers. These centers were taught how to operate collaboratives in their local geographies and effectively acted as franchises—we did not employ them. This meant we could have 10 waves operating simultaneously. No practice was counted as a spread site unless it produced monthly data. In 44 months—by December 2004—we engaged with almost 5,000 practices covering 32 million patients in England and achieved 72% improvement in access and a fourfold-greater reduction in mortality from CHD in the early waves than the rest of England. (I say the "early waves" because the subsequent activity covered most of England, and the differential disappeared.) The creation of the infrastructure and the cohort of clinicians and others familiar with improvement science meant that we could (and did) repeat the exercise with other topics, such as diabetes and chronic obstructive airway disease. For any given topic, we could have every part of England working on it within nine months. The full story is related in *The Small Book About Large System Change*.[3]

My colleagues and I have applied the knowledge of how to conduct a successful spread initiative to a variety of topics and in a variety of settings. For example, I assisted in developing the Primary Care Collaborative across Australia, with equivalent results to what we achieved in England. Beyond health care, we conducted collaboratives to increase the achievement of boys in schools in England and, with members of economically deprived communities as team members, to raise "social capital" by achieving improvement in nutrition and falls in older people. The situations and challenges are varied, but the spread method is generic.

If you follow the road map laid out in the Framework for Spread and apply methods and lessons from the case studies—and achieve systemwide change—then you will bring along a culture change in its wake. I have seen this happen several times. In England, general practices took on board the measurement of the quality of care as part of their remuneration, and in Australia, the collaborative brought about changes in governmental policy to facilitate teamwork and enhanced nurse roles. For example, whereas payment had only been provided for physician-provided care, payment for chronic disease care was now given for team-provided care. In this book, the case studies on Beth Israel Medical Center and Ascension Health both address the culture change engendered by the large-scale improvement effort. This leads me to the last and most crucial point, which comes through in all the case studies—and reflects my own experience: You cannot mandate the changes you want. In our case, we were dealing with thousands of independent businesses in general practice, just as several of the spread efforts described in the case studies in this book had to deal with local autonomy. The psychology and social aspects of the change process are critical—perhaps more so than anything else. Systemwide change, no matter how large the system, is about winning hearts and minds.

The time for projects and initiatives is over. The time is upon us to go to scale for what we already know. Our patients deserve nothing less. We owe Kevin Nolan and Marie Schall and and the other contributors to the book for showing us so expertly how to do that.

References

1. Rogers E.: *Diffusion of Innovations,* 4th ed. New York City: The Free Press, 1995.
2. Gladwell M.: *The Tipping Point: How Little Things Can Make a Big Difference.* New York City: Little, Brown and Company, 2000.
3. Oldham J.: *Sic Evenit Ratio Ut Componitur: The Small Book About Large System Change.* Marsh Lane, U.K.: Kingsham Press, 2004.

Introduction

Why Spread?

If you have recently been to a sports event or family occasion such as a graduation or wedding, there's a good chance that you have seen someone pull out a cell phone and snap a picture—or that you have snapped one yourself. Although cell phones have become almost universal, the ability to take pictures with a phone and then send them over the Internet to friends and relatives is relatively new. At first, the camera feature was optional on the higher-priced phones, so consumers had to make a conscious decision to buy one with that feature. The cost of the phone had to be weighed against the desirability of the new feature. Was it easy to use? How often would one want to take pictures? Was the quality of the pictures any good? These are the kinds of decisions that early adopters make when considering purchasing a new piece of technology or considering a change in behavior.

The diffusion of this new technology was helped along by the cell phone companies' decision to make the camera feature standard on all moderately priced cell phones. If only the spread of good ideas and practices in health care were so easy. An extensive literature has examined various aspects of this issue. Several studies that have examined this issue, including changing physician behavior and practices, provide some insight. Physician knowledge and attitudes about specific changes,[1,2] concerns about the associated costs of new processes or treatments,[3] and the reputation of the source of the new knowledge[4,5] are all factors that contribute to the rate of spread in health care. In addition, the delivery of health care is complex and often involves the coordination of large numbers of health care professionals, information, and equipment—not to mention the patients themselves. Another factor that may affect the spread of innovations is that the improvements intended for wider adoption are quite frequently *operational systems*—processes and related resources that support the basic functions of the organization—rather than discrete drugs or pieces of equipment. Extensive marketing methods are used to encourage the use of new medications. However, no such methods exist to support the spread of a new process to reliably order, dispense, and administer drugs safely within a hospital or to ensure that patients with diabetes are up to date on their recommended blood tests or eye exams.

These are the challenges. However, there are methods that health care providers and their organizations can use to spread good ideas and practices more easily and quickly. Using default features, as was done with cell phone cameras, is one such method. This book, *Spreading Improvement Across Your Health Care Organization,* is about those methods—the science and practice of spread as applied to health care.

We Know It Can Be Done

Six years ago, the Institute of Medicine issued its challenge in *Crossing the Quality Chasm*[6]; health care today is still not as good as it could be. What is holding back the health care system? It cannot be a lack of good intentions, efforts, or even examples of dramatically better systems.

Rather, it is the fact that better ideas and practices that are adopted by individuals or organizations are not always effectively shared with others. Donald Berwick has suggested several promising approaches for disseminating innovation, including finding and supporting innovators, investing in early adopters who are willing to try new ideas and making their actions visible to others, enabling reinvention, and providing time and resources to support the development of new ideas.[7] The Framework for Spread, which provides the conceptual backbone for this book, builds on these ideas and offers individuals and organizations guidance on how to organize themselves to accelerate the spread of ideas that are ready for broad dissemination.

The Institute for Healthcare Improvement's 5 Million Lives Campaign has applied effective concepts and strategies for spread in its linkage of thousands of hospitals' efforts to reduce the number of incidents of harm to patients. The campaign has shown that good ideas and practices can be made available and spread rapidly among large numbers of providers and organizations.[8] Two of the case study chapters in this book describe successful efforts to spread the campaign interventions. The story of the rapid and extensive spread of improved access and optimal care for persons with cardiovascular disease and other conditions by the National Primary Care Development Team in the United Kingdom, as described by Sir John Oldham in the Foreword, expands our vision of what can be accomplished using common strategies—even within a health care system with a delivery system and payment structure very different from those of the United States. We can learn from these and the examples in the other case study chapters on how to accelerate spread within our organizations and communities so that more and more patients will receive safer and better care.

Building an Improvement Infrastructure

The capability to spread improvements within an organization is an important aspect of a well-developed improvement infrastructure. Yet changes are not likely to spread if changes do not improve performance or the new levels of performance are not sustained over time. Therefore, an improvement infrastructure also includes the following:

- **The capability to make improvements.** Making improvements includes local incremental improvement and fundamental redesign of systems of care. Improvement frameworks such as the Model for Improvement[10] are useful for setting up projects and testing changes to improve performance.

- **The capability to implement successful changes.** *Implementation* refers to making successful changes part of the day-to-day operations so the gains are sustained. Some principles to consider when implementing changes are as follows:
  — Document the standard process
  — Make necessary changes to job descriptions (within scope of practice)
  — Assign ownership
  — Use measurement and audits to assure adherence to the standard process

Any organization that is committed to improvement will need to constantly improve the three capabilities of making, implementing, and spreading improvement.

Who Needs to Know About Spread?

This book is intended for anyone who wants to contribute to or even lead the spread of good ideas and practices in their organizations or communities in an effort to accelerate improvement. It explains the important role that a physician, a nurse, or another frontline caregiver can play in developing the initial improvements that others can adopt in their own settings. Middle managers will find guidance on how to support their units and departments in testing and implementing new ideas or practices. If you are a senior leader within your organization, the book will help you develop a plan to lead spread by setting an agenda for change, designating responsibility, and staying connected to the ongoing work. It especially addresses the role of the day-to-day leaders of the spread process, including responsibilities and key activities that contribute to successful spread efforts.

If you are experienced with improvement and have tested and implemented new ideas and practices at one or two sites within your organization, this book will help you develop a plan for moving those ideas and practices to other parts of your organization. Those who are new to improvement will learn how to establish the foundation for spread even while beginning improvements in a local area.

How to Use This Book

Chapter 1, "A Framework for Spread," presents an overall conceptual approach to spread and introduces a framework that organizes the components that have been shown to contribute to successful spread into a coherent whole. Practical guidance is provided throughout the chapter to assist the reader in applying the theory and methods of spread to his or her organization.

The case studies in the subsequent chapters provide examples of successful spread strategies and methods:

- Ascension Health System: Changes in practice that reduced pressure ulcers in a large health care system

- Beth Israel Medical Center: A set of prescribed processes that reduced central line infections and central line–associated bloodstream infections in two hospitals in an academic setting

- Kaiser Permanente: A system called Nurse Knowledge Exchange that improved efficiency and quality of patient care at shift change on nursing units across a large hospital system

- New York City Health and Hospitals Corporation: A redesigned system for chronic illness care in the ambulatory clinics of a large urban public health system that improved the quality of patient care

- The National Vascular Access Improvement Initiative (which became known as the "Fistula First" initiative): Use of a native arterial venous fistula as the preferred type of vascular access for hemodialysis by the 18 End-Stage Renal Disease (ESRD) networks across the United States

We appreciate the efforts of all persons involved in the work described in the case studies. They have made great contributions not only to the patients and staff in their organizations but also to the theory and practice of spreading improvement.

Chapter 7, "Insights and Conclusions," offers commentary and reflections on the case studies and highlights the lessons learned for other organizations engaging in spread.

We are pleased to present our best knowledge about how to spread good ideas and practices, which can be applied to virtually any health care organization and to community, regional, national, and even global improvement initiatives.

Many persons and organizations have contributed to the learning that resulted in the approach to spread described in this book. Fabiane Erb of VISN 2 of the Veterans Health Administration, Gail Nielsen of Iowa Health System, and John Whittington, M.D., formerly of OSF Health System, deserve special acknowledgement for their successful spread work within their organizations. We also acknowledge the global spread work of M. Rashad Massoud, M.D., and his contribution to the principles in Chapter 1 that guide the development of a spread plan.

References

1. Cabana M., et al.: Why don't physicians follow clinical practice guidelines? A framework for improvement. *JAMA* 282:1458–1465, Oct. 20, 1999.
2. Schuster R.J., et al.: Changing physician practice behavior to measure and improve clinical outcomes. *Am J Med Qual* 21:394–400, Nov.–Dec. 2006.
3. Grimshaw J.M., et al.: Changing physicians' behavior: What works and thoughts on getting more things to work. *J Contin Educ Health Prof* 22:237–243, Fall 2002.
4. Lomas J., et al.: Opinion leaders vs audit and feedback to implement practice guidelines: Delivery after previous cesarean section. *JAMA* 265:2202–2207, May 1, 1991.
5. Lomas J.: The in-between world of knowledge brokering. *BMJ* 334:129–132, Jan. 20, 2007.
6. Institute of Medicine: *Crossing the Quality Chasm: A New Health System for the 21st Century.* Washington, DC: National Academy Press, 2001.
7. Berwick D.M.: Disseminating innovations in health care. *JAMA* 289:1969–1975, Apr. 16, 2003.
8. McCannon C.J., et al.: Saving 100,000 lives in U.S. hospitals. *BMJ* 332:1328–1330, Jun. 3, 2006.
9. McCannon C.J., Hackbarth A.D., Griffin F.A.: Miles to go: An introduction to the 5 Million Lives Campaign. *Jt Comm J Qual Patient Saf* 33:477–484, Aug. 2007.
10. Langley G.J., et al.: *The Improvement Guide.* San Francisco: Jossey-Bass, 1996.

Chapter 1
A Framework for Spread

Kevin M. Nolan, M.A.
Marie W. Schall, M.A.

In 2000, the Institute for Healthcare Improvement (IHI) began testing approaches to spread projects in health care, as others did in other industries. Figure 1-1 (page 2) presents the Framework for Spread that evolved from that work. It is founded on Everett Rogers's definition of diffusion—"a process by which new ideas are communicated over time through a social system"[1 (p. 5)]—and draws both from the literature, including social learning theory,[2] social marketing,[3] and the theory of self-change,[4] and our experience. The framework is based on the belief that it is the individuals throughout an organization who play the leading role in the decision as to whether to adopt a "new idea"—that is, change their behaviors. The role of leadership, which sets the agenda, is to help them understand the need to improve performance and to support the spread activities.

The Framework for Spread identifies key components to consider when developing and executing a spread strategy—including leadership, the organizational "set-up" to support spread, the description of the new or better ideas, methods of communication, nurturing of the social system, measurement and feedback systems, and knowledge management. The framework is not prescriptive. Rather, its components suggest general areas for a team or an organization to consider in undertaking a spread project. The key components of the framework are as follows:

- The *Leadership* component of the framework should be considered a prerequisite to undertaking a large spread project within an organization. Bold aims for improvement require strong leadership support. Senior leaders (for example, the chief executive officer, the chief operating officer, the chief medical officer, the chief nursing officer) set the agenda. Facility leaders and middle managers, both clinical and administrative, need to align their priorities with the organizational agenda and encourage and assist staff in making the necessary changes. A special leadership role falls to an executive sponsor. The executive sponsor is the leader in the organization who is responsible and accountable for improved performance from the spread initiative and, therefore, is more directly involved with planning and executing the spread plan.

- How the ideas are described as part of the *Better Ideas* component of the framework, and their benefit relative to other ideas, will influence their rate of spread.

- The elements contained in the *Set-up* component form the foundation for the spread strategy. For example, understanding the size of the target population and the different audiences (for example, clerks, nurses, and physicians) will affect the communication plan.

Figure 1-1.
FRAMEWORK FOR SPREAD

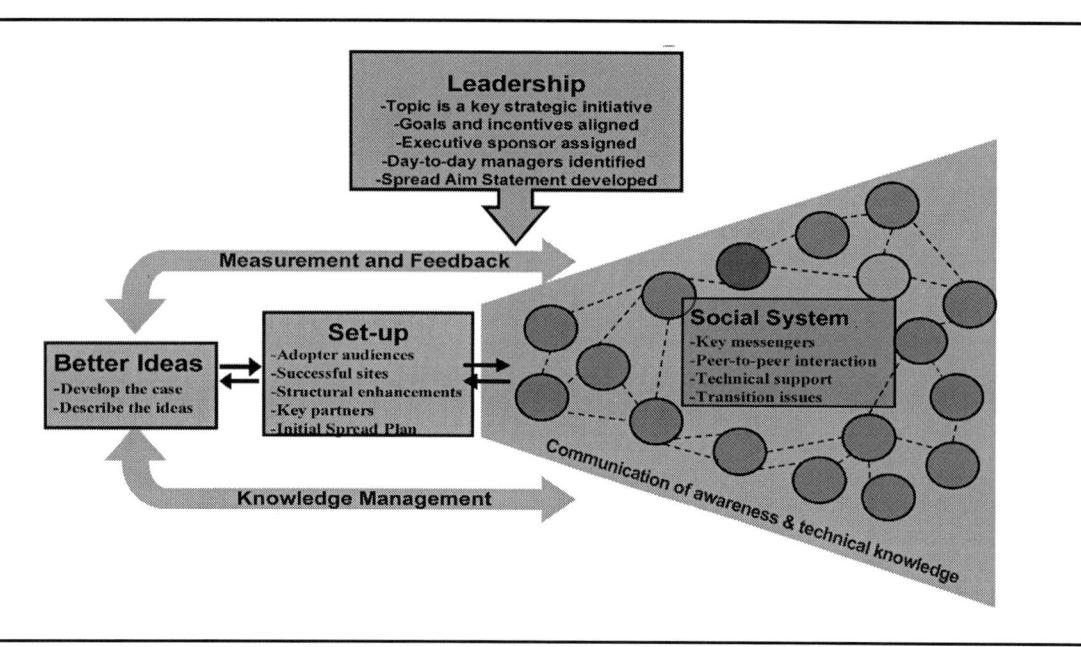

Leadership
- Topic is a key strategic initiative
- Goals and incentives aligned
- Executive sponsor assigned
- Day-to-day managers identified
- Spread Aim Statement developed

Measurement and Feedback

Better Ideas
- Develop the case
- Describe the ideas

Set-up
- Adopter audiences
- Successful sites
- Structural enhancements
- Key partners
- Initial Spread Plan

Social System
- Key messengers
- Peer-to-peer interaction
- Technical support
- Transition issues

Knowledge Management

Communication of awareness & technical knowledge

The Framework for Spread, developed by the Institute for Healthcare Improvement, identifies key components to consider when developing and executing a spread strategy.

- The *Social System* component suggests elements to strengthen connections within the system to facilitate spread. Communication is the foundation. Adopters must first be aware of the purpose of the spread initiative and then be spurred to action through interaction with others.

- *Measurement and Feedback* and *Knowledge Management* systems, which are used to monitor progress and serve as input to improve the strategy, are essential components of successful spread.

Using the Framework for Spread

A number of organizations have improved system performance by spreading ideas using the Framework for Spread.[5–7] For example, the Veterans Health Administration (VHA) used the framework to achieve a key strategic objective to improve patient access to care. The initiative involved more than 1,800 outpatient clinics between April 2001 and December 2003.[8,9] As a result, the waiting time for a primary care appointment within the VHA's 21 Veterans Integrated Service Networks (VISNs) decreased from an average of 60.4 days at the end of fiscal year (FY) 2000 to 28.4 at the end of FY 2002, with few resources being added.

One of the VISNs involved in the spread initiative was the VA Healthcare Network of Upstate New York (VISN 2). VISN 2 consists of 5 medical centers and 27 community-based outpatient clinics. Senior leaders within VISN 2 made improvement in patient access to care a key priority. They established a multifunctional steering committee or spread team and appointed VISN and medical center points of contact to manage the day-to-day activities of the spread strategy. VISN 2's spread team developed and carried out a communication plan to raise awareness and assist individuals to make changes. The VHA assembled an easy-to-use booklet that describes the key ideas to improve access, which was posted on the national VHA Web site. Because of the succinct packaging of the better ideas, clinics could readily test changes. VISN 2 shared the ideas in waves of face-to-face meetings. Relationships developed among physicians, nurses, and schedulers through dialogues at these meetings and visits to facilities. The spread team communicated and celebrated the success of adopters, resulting in a positive effect on participation. Waiting times for primary care patients in VISN 2 decreased from an average of more than 50 days in April 2001 to fewer than 20 days in 2003—results that have been sustained. Through the continued efforts in VISN 2, the waiting times in FY 2004 averaged approximately 16 days.

To use the Framework for Spread to develop and execute a spread strategy as the VHA did, it is helpful to consider the framework in terms of three connected phases:

> Determining organizational readiness for spread
> ↓
> Developing an initial spread plan
> ↓
> Executing and refining the spread plan

The sections that follow explain the phases, which are represented together in the Spread Work Plan and Time Line (Appendix 1-1, page 22) in some detail.

Determining Organizational Readiness for Spread
1. The topic is a key strategic objective
2. Executive sponsorship
3. Day-to-day manager
4. Spread team
5. Availability of ideas others will adopt

Senior leaders must make the decision as to whether the organization is ready to undertake a *spread initiative*—that is, undertake an initiative to foster widescale adoption of new ideas in practice to improve organizational performance. Leaders can use the following list to help determine whether an organization is ready for spread:

- The topic is connected to a key strategic objective.
- An executive sponsor is responsible and accountable.
- A capable day-to-day manager has been assigned.
- A spread team is created to assist the executive sponsor and the day-to-day manager.
- The case for improvement and a description of the ideas are available from successful sites.

1. The Topic Is a Key Strategic Objective. When an organization conducts strategic planning (usually yearly), it identifies objectives, develops a plan to achieve those objectives, and assigns resources to implement the plan. For a spread initiative to have a reasonable chance for success, senior leaders must make the topic (for example, improved access to primary care, reduced adverse events in a hospital) one of the organization's limited number of key strategic objectives.

A topic could also be an important means to achieve an objective. For example, an organization might identify improved access to primary care as one of a few means to achieve the objective of increasing revenue.

Once an organization identifies the topic of the spread initiative as a key strategic objective, senior leaders, along with facility leaders and middle managers, should support the work through the following activities[10]:

- Align systemwide and local goals and incentives with the spread aim. This may require changes to an organization's reward and recognition systems. For example, if the initiative involves key skills, human resources may need to develop tools to measure and develop those skills and, perhaps, make review of the skills a part of the annual appraisal system.

- Review and comment on the initial plan for spread. (Further discussion on what should be considered as part of a spread plan is presented in the sections that follow.)

- Assist with crafting an engaging and compelling message rather than mandating involvement.

- Schedule regular attention to review progress and provide advice.

- Be visible; for example, visit the units where improvements are being made.

- Use two-way communication with staff to gain knowledge about the work of the frontline teams and reinforce the importance of their efforts.

- Assign great performers to the effort; make improvement an important part of the job, not added work.

- Provide progress reports to the board.

2. Executive Sponsorship. Senior leaders should designate an executive sponsor to be responsible and accountable for the work and the results of the spread initiative. This person should have some connection to the areas (for example, outpatient services, medical-surgical units) where the new ideas will be spread and have the authority to make decisions about the changes. The executive sponsor's role should include the following activities:

- Play an active role in the development of the spread plan.

- Support the activities needed to achieve results, including assistance in overcoming barriers.

- Monitor progress and assist in revising the spread plan, as needed.

- Keep the initiative current; that is, continually help other leaders, middle managers, and staff understand the importance of the initiative in the organization's day-to-day work.

The executive sponsor plays a very important dual role. He or she is both a coach to the spread team and a "sense maker" to others in the organization to ensure alignment and support for the efforts. The executive sponsor should keep the initiative front and center during regularly scheduled meetings and through other existing communication channels within the organization.

3. Day-to-Day Manager. Senior leaders should select and give authority to a person to manage the day-to-day spread activities. The day-to-day manager's role is to assist potential adopters to make decisions consistent with the organization's strategic direction. He or she organizes and drives the work—and needs to work effectively with the executive sponsor. Depending on the structure and size of the organization, the day-to-day manager may have assistants to help manage the work in different regions or other segments within the organization.

It is useful if the day-to-day manager has good problem-solving and improvement skills (related to making, implementing, and spreading improvements) and is familiar with the topic that is the focus of the initiative. He or she should also be able to pay attention to detail but tolerate uncertainty, get along well with people, understand the culture and structure of the organization well, be passionate about the topic, and not require constant recognition.[11] The day-to-day manager's role is detailed in terms of the activities shown in Table 1-1 (page 7).

4. Spread Team. The spread team should assist the executive sponsor and the day-to-day manager in achieving the spread initiative's goals. The executive sponsor oversees the team, and the day-to-day manager is the team leader. The executive sponsor and the day-to-day manager select the team, on the basis of the expertise needed, with approval from senior leadership. Candidates should be allowed to make the decision as to whether to become members of the team. The executive sponsor and the day-to-day manager should negotiate the time necessary to be on the team with a candidate's supervisors, which could vary from a few hours a month to a few hours a week. Depending on the ideas being spread, team members should represent several areas of expertise and responsibility—line- or department-level representation from the areas affected; clinical expertise; representatives of a successful site; assistants to the day-to-day managers; and support services, such as information technology, human resources, and quality improvement. One individual may have expertise in more than one area. The size and composition of the spread team may vary, depending on the size of the organization and the complexity of the changes being spread. Examples of spread teams are provided in Sidebar 1-1 (page 5).

5. Availability of Ideas Others Will Adopt. When a spread initiative is started, an important first step for the spread team is gathering and describing the key ideas to be spread. This step is easiest if a package of evidence-based changes already exists, such as the Chronic Care Model (see Chapter 5) or the central line bundle (see Chapter 3). If such a package does not exist, the spread team can gather ideas by reviewing the literature and observing and meeting

Sidebar 1-1.
EXAMPLES OF SPREAD TEAMS FOR INITIATIVES FOCUSED ON IMPROVING PATIENT SAFETY AND IMPROVING ACCESS IN PHYSICIAN OFFICES AND CLINICS

1. Patient Safety—Small System (e.g., within 1 hospital)
   Executive sponsor: Vice president of medical affairs
   Day-to-day manager: Patient safety officer
   Other members of the team:
   - The team leader from a successful unit
   - Representatives of the nurse managers of the target units

2. Patient Safety—Large System (e.g., 15-hospital system)
   Executive sponsor: Corporate vice president of medical affairs
   Day-to-day manager: Corporate patient safety officer (assistants: patient safety officers at the hospitals)
   Other members of the team:
   - The team leader from a successful site
   - A pharmacist, nurse manager, risk manager, or quality officer from each of the target hospitals

3. Access in Physician Offices and Clinics—Small System (e.g., 6 sites)
   Executive sponsor: Medical director
   Day-to-day manager: Director/practice manager (with technical expertise in improving access)
   Other members of the team:
   - A physician and nurse (and/or other team members) from the pilot clinic
   - Representatives of the practice managers from the target sites
   - Representatives of the clinical leaders of the target sites

4. Access in Physician Offices and Clinics—Large System (e.g., 50–60 sites in four regions)
   Executive sponsor: Chief medical officer
   Day-to-day manager: Director of service performance for the system (with technical expertise in improving access); assistants in the regions
   Other members of the team:
   - A physician and nurse manager (and/or other team members) from the pilot clinic
   - The clinic administrator/director responsible for each region
   - A clinician from each region

with representatives from successful sites both within and outside the organization. *Successful sites are those that have achieved high performance in the topic that is the focus of the spread initiative.*

In describing the ideas, the spread team should keep in mind the five key attributes that Rogers[1] identified as influencing the rate of spread of ideas:

- Relative advantage over other ideas to achieve the desired outcome

- Compatibility with existing values, experiences, and needs

- Complexity that could inhibit an adopter's ability to understand and use the ideas

- Trialability that allows ideas to be tried on a small scale and reversed if desired

- Observability of the ideas in practice.

Table 1-2 (page 7) is a worksheet based on these attributes, which the spread team can use to assess the likelihood that their ideas will spread. The spread team can assess the ideas as a group or individually.

In Rogers's view, the relative advantage of the changes is the most important attribute.[1] Bandura[2] also highlights the importance of relative advantage to move people to change behavior. Most persons are attracted to ideas that make their work easier and also benefit patients/customers. When new ideas are simply added to existing work, they are often resisted as creating a burden rather than a benefit. The spread team should ask the question "Do the employees most affected by the change understand the reason for it and believe it is worthwhile?" They should also ask "What is the percentage of increased effort that employees must make to implement the changes?" Optimally, employees should experience less than 10% extra work to test the new ideas and a positive impact on work load once the new ideas are implemented.[11]

Senior leaders also need to weigh the advantages of the new ideas with the business case, especially if structural changes are needed within the organization to support the new system.

Organizations often ask, "When are ideas ready for spread?" This is a decision most readily made by adopters. Not everyone will adopt new ideas at the same time. Spread starts slowly and gains momentum. The spread team should focus on communicating the work of the successful sites using Rogers's five key attributes of new ideas. If the ideas rate reasonably high on the attributes, adopters should be attracted to the work.

Successful sites that exist when the spread initiative starts are important contributors to the description of the ideas being spread. To continue to attract others to adopt the ideas, additional sites within the organization need to achieve results by testing and implementing the ideas gathered and described. The day-to-day manager and executive sponsor should focus their early work to develop such sites. They should make this an opportunity for learning by understanding how the ideas are adapted to the new setting, what transition issues are faced, and the factors (for example, leadership support, adherence to schedules) that affect the pace of improvement.

If adoption of the ideas is not gaining momentum over time, the spread team should attempt to strengthen the rating of the new ideas on the five attributes. It should also closely study the units within the target population that *are not* achieving the results predicted and amend the description of the changes, as necessary, on the basis of the learning. The spread team might also learn about other barriers to improvement, such as the need for assistance with improvement methods or technical support.

Bandura[2] suggests the use of incentives to attract people to the work in the early stages of a spread initiative. The spread team could indeed use external motivators to spur involvement, especially early on, when the evidence about the benefits of new ideas or how to best test and implement them is often not yet fully developed. Examples of such motivators are protected time to accomplish the work, recognition, and appropriate privileges (for example, first choice of work schedules, ability to work from home). As learning about the ideas and their benefits increases, the spread team can more readily count on increased motivation and momentum resulting from the ability of adopters to more quickly achieve improved performance.

Although organizations can bring about improvement through widescale adoption of new ideas, senior leaders should also consider changes that might be needed in the organization's structure. *Structure* is the basic configuration of an organization that affects how the components connect or interact.[12] Changes in structure such as information technology, distribution channels, departments, and functions (for example, call centers) can play a large

Table 1-1.
ACTIVITIES FOR THE DAY-TO-DAY MANAGER

1. Oversee deployment of the spread plan:
   a. Connect with senior leaders, facility leaders, and middle managers to ensure their support
   b. Develop and manage a communication plan
   c. Support and leverage key messengers
   d. Identify successful sites to help make the case
   e. Package the ideas being spread
   f. Refine the spread plan with the support of the executive sponsor
2. Assist adopters to overcome transition issues:
   a. Listen for emerging issues
   b. Connect people who can assist one another in adopting the changes
   c. Share important issues with the appropriate leader
3. Report on progress and share learning:
   a. Be involved with the development of the measurement plan
   b. Track outcomes and the rate of spread. Make performance visible.
   c. Summarize/disseminate ongoing learning about the changes being made (knowledge management)

Table 1-2.
WORKSHEET TO ASSESS IDEAS FOR SPREAD

Key Ideas:

Attributes	Relative to the attribute, the ideas are					Comments
	Weak 1	2	Okay 3	4	Strong 5	
Relative advantage						
Compatibility with current system						
Simplicity						
Trialability						
Observability						

direct role in achieving the desired organizational outcomes or a supporting role in the spread of ideas. By making changes to and aligning fundamental structures in the organization to support the initiative, leaders signal the importance of the spread aim. Leveraging organizational structures to facilitate spread is a key consideration in the development of a spread plan and is discussed further later in this chapter.

When describing the ideas, the spread team should consider Rogers's attributes of complexity and trialability. That is, the team should describe the ideas in a succinct fashion and offer tips for adopters both on getting started and overcoming barriers. The description of ideas should give adopters confidence that they can make the changes while leaving room for adaptation at the local level.

Many operational systems, such as the system to improve patient access in outpatient clinics, are made up of multiple components. Therefore, in addition to describing the individual components and ideas, it is helpful to show how the components fit together (concept design). To make it easier to adapt the multiple components at the local level, the description might also suggest an optimal sequence for testing the ideas on the basis of the experience of successful sites. The work of the VHA,[9] as described earlier, can serve as an example of how to describe the key ideas to be spread (Sidebar 1-2, below).

Sidebar 1-2.
EXAMPLE OF DESCRIBING THE IDEAS TO BE SPREAD

To describe the ideas, the VHA spread team used a format that included a definition of the idea and some details on measures, tools and resources, tips, examples, and frequently asked questions. The concept design for the operational system to improve access is as follows:
- **Component 1:** Shape the demand.
- **Component 2:** Match capacity and demand.
- **Component 3:** Redesign the system to increase capacity.

As an example, consider the description of one idea, "Work Down the Backlog," for Component 1: Shape the demand.

Idea: Work Down the Backlog
Definition: "Backlog" consists of all appointments on the future schedule for a particular clinic. Bad backlog is work from previous days put off into the future. This backlog of appointments clogs clinic schedules, taking up slots that could be used for patients requesting appointments with their providers. Good backlog is necessary appointments scheduled to meet the needs of the patient in the future.

More Details: Work Down the Backlog

1. Measures to Use to Work Down the Backlog
Backlog can be measured in the following ways: number of patients scheduled or appointment slots filled. Start with today as the index day and look forward in the schedule. Not including today's appointments, count the total number of patients (or appointment slots) on the books. Go as far ahead in the schedule as there are appointments assigned to a patient. This can be done manually or electronically.

(continued)

Sidebar 1-2. (continued)
EXAMPLE OF DESCRIBING THE IDEAS TO BE SPREAD

Determine the percentage of future appointment slots filled: Select a particular time frame, such as 4 or 6 weeks from today. Count the total number of appointment slots (whether or not a patient has been assigned to the slots). This is your denominator. Now count the total number of appointment slots that are filled (a patient has been given an appointment for that time). This is your numerator. Compute the percentage of future appointment slots filled for the time period chosen. This can be done manually or electronically.

2. *Tools and Resources*
A tool such as one to calculate length of time needed to eliminate the backlog could be included here.

3. *Tips*
- Measure the extent of your backlog and make a plan for reducing your backlog.
- Use the scheduling system to generate a list of patients with multiple future appointments. Eliminate duplicate appointments that are not clinically appropriate.
- Don't allow the system to keep filling future appointments.
- Include clinic staff in making the plan to reduce your backlog.

4. *Examples*
- Include stories of how clinics worked down their backlogs; stories[9] discuss:
  — How big was the clinic's backlog
  — How it worked down its backlog
  — How long it took
  — Lessons learned

5. *Frequently Asked Questions*
Q: Once I've worked down my backlog, how do I prevent my appointment slots from being filled with other physicians' appointments or from being assigned new patients since I seem to have so much open time on my schedule?
A: There has to be a decision made by senior clinical and administrative leadership that physicians working on improving access will have a clearly defined panel and will be responsible only for their own patients once the appropriate panel size has been reached.

Q: Can I reduce my backlog by sending patients who want to be seen today to the urgent care clinic?
A: Sending overflow patients to urgent care actually adds to your backlog because, even if they go to the urgent care clinic, they will want to also come back to see their own provider. When this happens, they will be given an appointment in the future, thus adding to the backlog.

Q: Is the goal to have no backlog, so that there are no future appointments on our clinic schedules?
A: No. There will always be some backlog (the good backlog) on the schedule. Remember types of good backlog include (1) provider discretionary return appointments; (2) patient choice (patients call in today but want to come in tomorrow); and (3) automatic appointments at certain intervals to manage specific types of patients.

Developing an Initial Spread Plan
1. Developing an aim for spread
2. Developing an organizational structure for spread
3. Developing a communication plan
4. Developing a measurement plan for spread

1. Developing an Aim for Spread. If the leaders of an organization believe that they are ready to begin a spread initiative, they should start developing an aim for spread, which is an explicit statement that documents what the organization is to achieve in its spread effort. Examples of an aim statement for a spread initiative are provided in Sidebar 1-3 (page 11). Senior leaders, facility leaders, middle managers, and the spread team can use the aim statement to communicate the intent of the initiative throughout the organization. It will also guide the effort and keep it focused. Senior leaders should document the aim as part of strategic planning or assign the task to the executive sponsor and day-to-day manager. If the task is assigned, they should review and comment on the aim developed. In either case, an aim statement should include the following:

- The ideas, processes, or systems being spread (for example, system for improving access to primary care clinics, the components of the Chronic Care Model to improve diabetes care, a hospitalwide system to ensure patient safety, structural changes being considered to achieve the level of system improvement desired)

- The target population for spread (the units in your organization expected to adopt the new ideas or processes)

- The time frame for the spread activities (for example, within the next six months, within the next year)

- The target levels of system performance you want to achieve (for example, reduce the average glycosylated hemoglobin [A1C] levels for patients with diabetes to < 7.0, reduce adverse drug events in all medical and surgical units by 75%)

Once an organization finalizes its aim for spread, the spread team should begin to develop a plan to achieve it. Key components of a spread plan are a communication plan and a measurement plan. When a spread team is developing its plan, it will need to tailor elements of the Framework for Spread to meet its specific situation. For example, the organization's size and structure and existing communication channels and measurement capabilities will influence the plan. Considerations for developing a spread plan are discussed in some detail in this chapter. Tailoring the plan is evident in Chapters 2–6.

2. Developing an Organizational Structure for Spread. The strategy and tactics contained in a spread plan are influenced by an organization's structure. The following principles, many of which relate to organizational structure, guide the development of a spread plan:

- *Begin with full scale in mind.* The spread team should envision what the system would look like when a good percentage of the target population has adopted the ideas. Two considerations are as follows:

  — *Whether changes made in the initial site(s) are scalable.* For example, additional nursing hours or support from a health educator available at the initial spread site might not be available to all sites within the target population. The spread team should discuss the alternatives, keeping in mind the new work required and who could do it.

  — *The structural enhancements needed to support the new system at scale.* Ideas often cannot just be replicated from unit to unit but require support from enhanced organizational structures as they are spread. For example, to facilitate spread, multiple sites might need to be linked together electronically to share information, or scheduling systems might need to be improved. Key dimensions of structure to consider are how people are grouped together, the distribution of authority and accountability, physical structure (space design, equipment, capacity), and information technology capabilities. The spread team should take a proactive view of structural enhancements, which could make the transition to the new system easier for adopters and accelerate the rate of spread. Depending on the extent of the structural enhancements considered, senior leaders might need to be directly involved with these decisions.

Sidebar 1-3.
EXAMPLES OF AN AIM STATEMENT FOR A SPREAD INITIATIVE

1. **Patient Safety**
What We Intend to Spread: We will spread a safe, efficient, and effective medication system that includes the following key components:
- Executive walkarounds
- Unit briefings
- Reconciliation of medications
- Use of Failure Mode and Effects Analysis (FMEA)
- A focus on high-hazard medications

Target Population and Time Frame for Spread (Small System): We will spread the new medication system from one medical-surgical unit to all inpatient units in our hospital in the next 18 months.

Or

Target Population and Time Frame for Spread (Large System): We will spread the new medication system to 35 hospitals in our system. In the next 12 months, we will spread to 10 hospitals in the same region as the successful hospital. In the second and third years of this spread effort, we will include the remaining 25 hospitals in our system.

Target Levels of System Performance: We will reduce adverse drug events (ADEs) in our hospital from an average of 30% of patients experiencing an ADE to < 5%.

2. **Medical-Surgical Units in a Hospital**
What We Intend to Spread: We will transform our hospital so that patients and their families receive patient-centered, safe, reliable, and value-added care from an empowered and supported care team. To reach this vision we will spread:
1. Multidisciplinary rounds (including setting daily goals)
2. Peace-and-quiet time on the nursing units
3. A nursing capacity/traffic light system
4. Rapid response teams
5. Scheduled discharges

Target Population and Time Frame: Within the next 18 months, we will spread the improvements listed above to all 10 patient care units in our hospital.

Target Levels of System Performance:
- Adverse events are reduced to ≤ 5 per 1,000 patient days
- 95% compliance with all key clinical process measures for the top three clinical conditions in nursing units
- 95% of patients report that they will recommend the hospital to family or friends
- Clinicians spend at least 70% of their time in direct patient care

- *In large organizations, take advantage of formal groupings in the organization.* The structural dimension of how units (for example, hospitals, clinics) are grouped together (for example, by region) is important in planning, especially in larger organizations. The VHA's division into 21 VISNs (as noted earlier) enabled the spread initiative on patient access to primary care to commence simultaneously in multiple regions. The regional authority plays a central role in managing the spread in its region. If formal groupings do not exist, the spread team can consider how artificial groupings might be established to allow for the spread initiative to commence in multiple areas in a large organization. It might consider the following questions about organizational groupings when developing a spread plan:

  — What is the geographic distribution of the units we want to spread to?

  — Where are the authority or influence centers?

  — How can we use the existing groupings within the organization to accelerate the rate of spread?

  — What groupings might be established to assist with spread?

- *If spread is to occur within a community, identify an entity to provide leadership.* Strong leadership is important if a spread project is to be successful. Often, leadership is not clearly defined at the outset and needs to be identified. For example, for a spread initiative focused on providing access to health care for the uninsured in a community such as Montgomery County, Maryland, certain entities (for example, state/local government, professional associations, the Quality Improvement Organization) might be able to provide leadership and gather and deploy resources. The identified entity would then need to enlist partners within the community that have a stake in the project to provide support.

- *Leverage the natural connections between sites in the target population.* Adopters will listen to those they know and respect, so existing relationships are powerful connectors in a social system. The spread team should first seek to understand these relationships, both formal and informal, through conversations with sites. It should then ensure that these connections are considered when the communication plan is developed. For example, the spread team could arrange a visit to a high-performing site by potential adopters who have a relationship with staff at that site.

- *Plan to use members of successful sites as coaches for spread.* As part of an initial spread plan, the spread team should identify persons to assist in raising awareness and providing technical support. It should consider representatives from successful sites on the basis of their influence with others, communication skills, and knowledge of the ideas being spread. The spread team members must manage the site representatives' time commitments and consider developing the representatives' skills in coaching and improvement.

- *Consider both completeness and coverage.* The ideas being spread may have multiple major components. For example, the concept design for improving patient access to care has these components: shape the demand, match capacity and demand, and redesign the system to increase capacity.[9] One approach could be to focus on the spread of one component initially, such as shaping demand—that is, provide "coverage" of the target population with part of the ideas. Alternatively, an organization might focus on the adoption of all the components (completeness) by a few sites initially. Obviously, many different combinations of completeness and coverage are possible. When including a certain approach in an initial spread plan, an organization should consider the following[13]:

  — *The impact:* What approach will result in the largest benefits early on so others can be attracted to the work?

  — *Resources:* What approach will maximize the use of available resources?

  — *Interdependence:* Which ideas are considered foundational to the adoption of the other ideas? Can these ideas be adopted independently of the others and still work?

— *Learning:* What are the important things that need to be learned? For example, a coverage approach might be considered if it is important to learn whether a key change, such as the use of a care team in primary care, can work across different environments in the target population.

— *Path of least resistance:* Is there support throughout the organization for the new ideas, or is support only in certain areas? Are there other initiatives going on in the organization that could support or hinder involvement at certain sites? Is geography an issue in achieving coverage?

- *Develop partnerships.* Organizations should consider forming mutually beneficial partnerships that could contribute to the success of the project. These partnerships could be with entities within the organization, such as union representatives or ancillary departments, or outside the organization, such as professional associations or government entities. Partners can support the communication of the initiative and its benefits. Before partnerships can be forged, the spread team should listen to, understand, and address any issues pertaining to the project from potential partners.

3. Developing a Communication Plan. Because communication is at the heart of spread, a communication plan is an essential part of a spread plan. Developing and carrying out a communication plan is a central activity of the spread team. Prochaska, Norcross, and DiClemente suggest that adopters will progress through stages of change—from awareness to decision and from decision to action.[4] The spread team should consider the communication tactics, including the messages, needed to assist the adopter in making the transition between these stages. Because part of the target population will be in each stage of change throughout most of the spread initiative, tactics for the different stages will be an ongoing part of an organization's communication plan.

- *From awareness to decision.* Because individuals must perceive they have a problem before they are willing to change behavior, the spread team should first begin a communication campaign[14] to raise awareness about the extent of the problem and the benefits of change.[15] Consistent with social marketing, the team should tailor the message to the different segments of potential adopters (for example, clinicians, schedulers, administrators) and should communicate the following information:

— Patient and staff stories that illuminate the extent of the problem

— Feedback (data) to adopters on performance

— Benefits for each segment of adopters

— General overview of the new ideas

— Frequently asked questions about the ideas

The method of communication is also important. Spread teams can use general communication (for example, flyers, newsletters), methods that can convey a more personal touch (for example, letters, cards) or interactive methods (for example, e-mail, telephone).[16]

A spread team can adapt the worksheet provided as Table 1-3 (page 19) to document its communication plan to raise awareness. The example contained in the table is based on an organization's spread of ideas to improve access to primary care. It includes the plan for two adopter segments, clinicians and receptionists. A complete plan would also include other adopter segments, such as medical assistants and call center staff.

The spread team should develop a plan to monitor whether the communication campaign is working. On the basis of the time frame included in the organization's aim for spread, the spread team should define measurable objectives for outcomes of the campaign (for example, percentage of the target population that should make the decision to adopt within three months, six months, and so on). Monitoring the communication plan, including questions the spread team might ask if milestones are not met, is discussed later in this chapter.

- *From decision to action.* Once individuals make the decision to adopt, they are more inclined to listen to technical knowledge about the ideas. Knowledge about the ideas goes beyond the "what" to the "how to" for adapting the ideas. To facilitate moving adopters from decision to action, the spread team must ensure that its plan includes communication methods that allow adopters to interact with their colleagues. Avorn and Soumerai[17] discuss the benefits of person-to-person contact in educational outreach. Szulanski and Winter[18] suggest visits to high-performing sites to aid in replication of best practices. Wegner, McDermott, and Snyder[19] describe the benefits of bringing together groups of individuals with like jobs and interests to form communities of practice.

  The size of the organization plays a role in the communication methods used to move potential adopters to action and how those methods are deployed. The VHA used a series of nationally sponsored meetings to foster peer-to-peer interaction and facilitate the development of successful sites in each of its networks. When successful sites were developed, the VHA used its network structure to accelerate spread. Each network developed its own communication plan to allow adopters to interact. These plans included methods such as meetings, mentoring, and visits.

  As the spread team shares content knowledge, adopters will often need additional help and support to successfully adapt the changes to their local areas. The spread team should ensure that such technical support, which persons at sites successful at adopting the changes can provide, is available.

- *Messengers.* As the spread team develops its communication plan, it must identify and recruit messengers to assist the team. Persons who are influencers or opinion leaders in the social system serve as the best messengers.[20–22] Asking potential adopters, "Who do you go to for advice on a particular topic?" can help identify opinion leaders. Opinion leaders who can influence the spread process are usually peers of the potential adopters and, therefore, often frontline staff rather than managers. When the spread team is enlisting and using opinion leaders as messengers, it should do the following:

  — Be careful not to overly formalize the role of an opinion leader and thereby disrupt this informal leadership position.

  — Pay attention to opinion leaders who do not support the spread initiative. Not all opinion leaders will be early adopters of the changes being spread. It is worth taking the time to understand and address the issues of those who are not.

  — Identify messengers with a high degree of content knowledge, whom Gladwell[23] calls "mavens." Mavens help supply the technical support needed by adopters. Do not assume, though, that messengers will be able to deliver succinct, easily understood information. Often, coaching of messengers is needed.

4. Developing a Measurement Plan for Spread. Measurement is an integral part of improvement. During a spread initiative, two different types of measures are useful: (1) measures that demonstrate the impact on system performance and (2) measures that demonstrate the extent of the spread of the new ideas. Because a spread project is focused on improving performance, the spread team should collect and plot data over time for the key outcome measure (for example, adverse drug events, time to third-next-available appointment in clinics, A1C levels for patients with diabetes). The team should include data from the target population identified in the spread aim. Iowa Health System developed a run chart that includes data from its 10 hospitals to monitor performance during its spread initiative (see Figure 1-2, page 15).

Along with the key outcome measures, an organization should also collect information on the rate of spread of the key ideas. Teams can gather this information by sampling from the target sites or from verbal reports. A more formal measurement system would have individual sites documenting (monthly) their progress from planning, to testing, to implementing on each of the key ideas. Iowa Health System uses the form shown in Figure 1-3 (page 16) to document

Figure 1-2.
PERCENTAGE OF SAMPLED CHARTS AT IOWA HEALTH SYSTEM WITH HARM LEVELS FOR ADVERSE DRUG EVENTS OF E–I, NOVEMBER 2001–JANUARY 2004

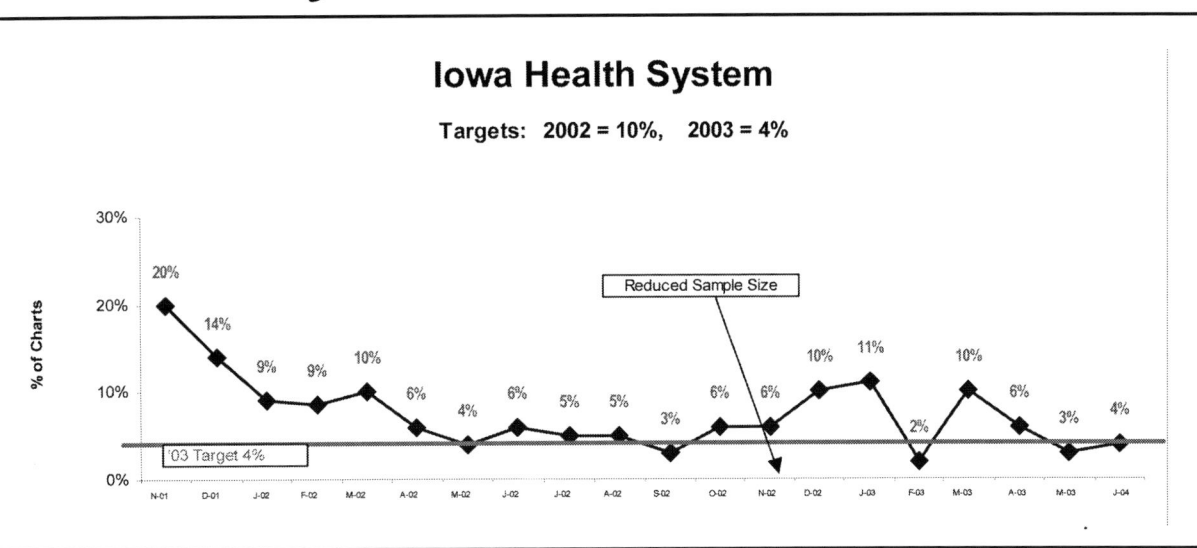

Iowa Health System developed this run chart, which includes data from the 10 hospitals in the system, to monitor performance during its spread initiative. According to the National Coordinating Council for Medication Error Reporting and Prevention (NCC MERP) Index for Categorizing Medication Errors, Categories E through I indicate patient harm (http://www.nccmerp.org/medErrorCatIndex.html [accessed Jul. 3, 2007]). Used with permission.

this progression. The spread team can plot over time the information collected on this form to depict the rate of spread of key ideas, as shown in Figure 1-4 (page 17).

Executing and Refining the Spread Plan
1. Communication of awareness
2. Identification of early adopters
3. Knowledge transfer and application by adopters
4. Feedback
5. Maintaining the gains

A spread team will find that spreading new ideas often does not go exactly as planned, so progress on the plan should be closely monitored as it is executed. The team can then provide the appropriate feedback to senior leaders, facility leaders, middle managers, and adopters. Adopters should receive feedback to assist them to make the transition through the stages of change—from awareness to decision and from decision to action. If these transitions are not going as planned, the spread team should provide leaders and managers with the information necessary to make adjustments to the spread plan.

When the plan is executed, the spread team should take an active role in "listening" to the target population to understand the issues getting in the way of adoption.[24] Adopters may be slow to adopt new ideas because of these transition issues and may need assistance to overcome them.[25] Issues might include, for example, the need for structural enhancements such as new equipment, adopters' understanding of the features of a new scheduling system, or a clinician's access to medical records. The spread team

Figure 1-3.
TRACKING THE SPREAD OF IDEAS AT IOWA HEALTH SYSTEM

A= Planning   B= Start   C= Testing In Progress   D= Fully Implemented

	Site 1				Site 2				Site 3				Site 4				Site 5			
	A	B	C	D	A	B	C	D	A	B	C	D	A	B	C	D	A	B	C	D
Steering Team				x				x		x						x	x			
Exec Walks				x				x				x				x		x		
Unit Briefings				x				x				x				x		x		
Medication FMEA				x				x				x				x	0			
Hazard Drug/Area # 1		x				x			x				x						x	
Hazard Drug/Area # 2	x					x			0				0				0			
Reconciliation		x				x			x					x					x	
Triggers and Alerts - ADEs			x			x					x				x					x
Issues Tracking Database			x			x				x					x					x
Patient Involvement	x				x				x				x				x			
Simulation		x			NA				NA				NA				NA			

Iowa Health System used this form to initially document sites' monthly progress from planning to start, testing, and implementing key ideas. Exec Walks, executive walkarounds; FMEA, Failure Mode and Effects Analysis; ADEs, adverse drug events. Used with permission.

should decide which issues need to be brought to the attention of management and which might be dealt with at the local level, perhaps by arranging a peer-to-peer discussion. The original successful sites are often helpful in identifying these barriers to adoption that, once addressed, can speed the spread of the new ideas to new sites. In fact, early on in the execution of the spread plan, when the evidence for the benefits of the changes is not fully developed, understanding and minimizing the transition issues is an important strategy to move adopters to action.[26]

1 and 2. Communication of Awareness and Identification of Early Adopters. Individuals in a social system do not adopt changes at the same time. On the basis of this temporal phenomenon, Rogers places adopters in categories from innovators to laggards.[1] Figure 1-5 (page 18) depicts the theoretical curve of the cumulative rate of adoption of a new idea. This theoretical curve is very similar to the curves shown in Figure 1-4 for the Iowa Health System. Rogers classifies approximately 15% of adopters as innovators or early adopters.

Gladwell refers to the point of acceleration in the curve as the *tipping point*.[23] Following the diffusion models developed by Bass[27] and referred to as the S curve, the tipping point has been shown to occur when the change has been adopted by 20% to 30% of the target population. At that point, a sufficient number of successful examples exist that the risks of adoption for others are lessened. This curve represents only the rate of adoption. As we know, adopters transition though stages of change, from awareness to decision to action. A more complete representation of the spread process is shown in Figure 1-6 (page 18), which also includes the cumulative rate of decision to adopt over time.

Figure 1-4.
DISPLAYING THE SPREAD OF IDEAS AT IOWA HEALTH SYSTEM, JANUARY 2001–NOVEMBER 2002

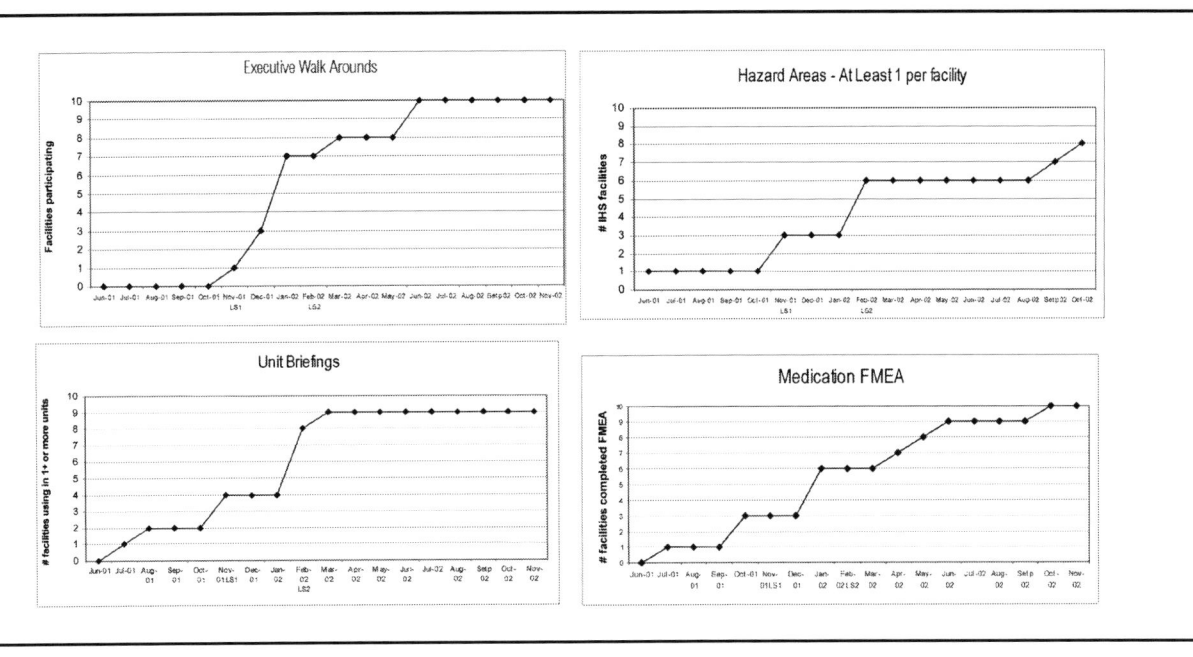

The information collected monthly, as shown in Figure 1-3, can be plotted over time to depict the rate of spread of key ideas through the 10 hospitals in the system. FEMA, Failure Mode and Effects Analysis. Used with permission.

The spread team should closely monitor the percentage of the target population who indicate that they will adopt the changes. For example, if an organization sets a two-year time frame to accomplish its spread goals, in the first six months, at least 15% of the target population should transition from awareness to making the decision to adopt the changes. This is based roughly on the S curves shown in Figure 1-6. If the identification of early adopters falls short of this marker, it should serve as a signal to the spread team and senior leaders to review and refine the spread plan. The following questions could be asked to assist in the review:

- Do the messages need improvement?

- How capable are the messengers?

- Are the communication methods effective? How many persons in the target population are aware of the spread initiative?

- Are there transition issues affecting those making the decision?

Early adopters are very important to the spread process. The spread team should actively listen to the target population to identify the early adopters, the activities that will move them to action, and the issues they raise. The spread team can integrate the successes of the early adopters into its communication plan and can use their learning to make it easier for the early and late majority to adopt the new ideas.

3. Knowledge Transfer and Application by Adopters. As adopters make the decision to adopt the changes, the spread team should execute the activities in its communication plan to help adopters take action. These activities include purposeful peer-to-peer interaction such as mentoring, visiting, and group discussions. Persons from successful sites can provide support to new adopters regarding

Figure 1-5.
THEORETICAL CURVE OF THE RATE OF ADOPTION

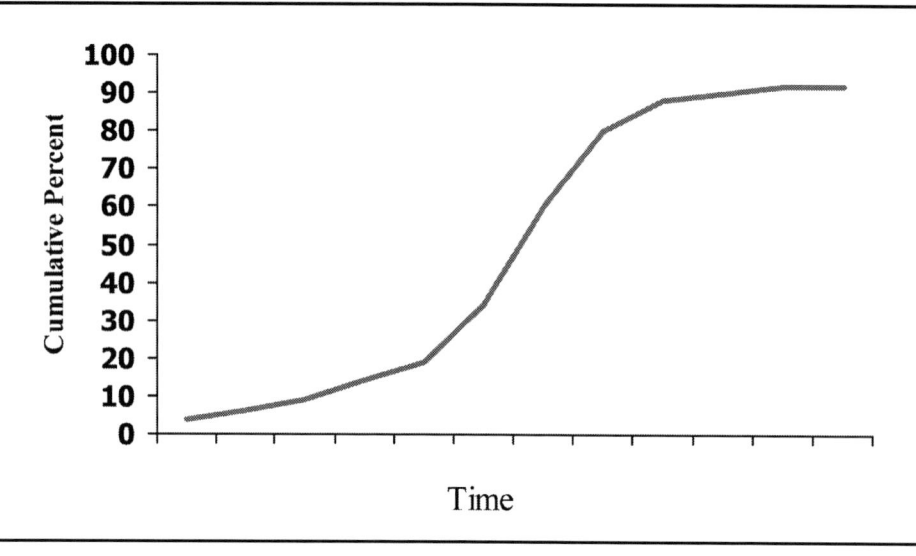

The theoretical curve of the cumulative rate of adoption of a new idea is shown. Adapted from Rogers E.: Diffusion of Innovations, *4th ed. New York City: The Free Press, 1995; and Bass F.: A new product growth model for consumer durables.* Management Science *13:215–227, Jan. 1969. Used with permission.*

Figure 1-6.
THEORETICAL CURVE OF THE RATE OF SPREAD

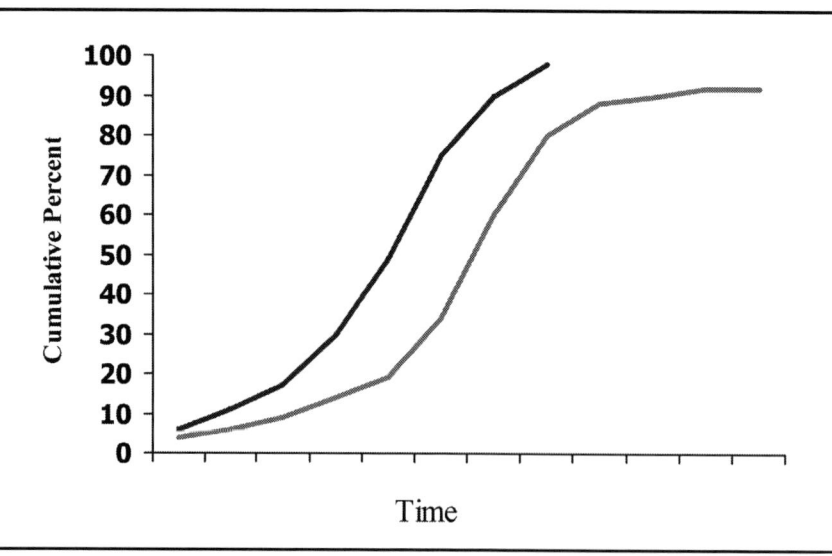

This more complete representation of the spread process includes the cumulative rate of decision to adopt (left) and the rate of adoption (right) over time. Adapted from the paper "Setting the Context for Change and Spread," by Van de Ven A.H.: Institute for Healthcare Improvement Spread Call to Action Series, Sep. 18, 2003. Used with permission.

Table 1-3.
WORKSHEET FOR COMMUNICATION OF AWARENESS

Audience	Messages	Tactics
Clinicians	- Take charge of your work life - See your own patients - Timelier care of patients	1. Use the newsletter and blast e-mails to convey the problem of long days for clinicians and long waits for patients 2. Share data on access and continuity with individual clinicians 3. Use conference calls to share success stories from clinicians and comments from patients
Receptionists	- More control of the day - Dealing with happier patients	Meeting for receptionists to discuss issues and benefits for them of improved access. Include success stories from receptionists and comments from patients.

the changes and overcoming transition issues. Adopters might also need quality improvement support to assist them in testing and implementing changes.

Most adopters will adapt new ideas to their situation. They may revise a form or change the way a certain self-management method is introduced to patients. Rogers refers to this as "reinvention." This active role of adopters in the spread process is a good thing. Not only will adopters optimize the ideas in their local setting, they will also add to the knowledge about the topic. The spread team should develop a system to capture the increasing knowledge base on an ongoing basis.[28] It might ask adopters to post new materials or refinements to the ideas to a Web site or visit sites to understand and document how the ideas were adapted. The new knowledge should make it easier for adopters in the future to make the changes.

As adopters move to action, senior leaders should judge the success of the spread initiative based on the outcome goals for the system documented in the aim for spread. They should request regular reports that include data on outcomes and on the progress of spread. In addition to aggregate data, the spread team will find data at the unit level very useful, especially early in the project. For example, in addition to monitoring adverse drug events at the system level, the spread team should monitor adverse drug events for individual hospitals identified as early adopters. It should be a clear signal to the spread team to conduct detailed reviews if units have done the following:

- Made the decision but are slow in actually making the changes and therefore show no improvement in outcomes

- Reported that they are making the changes but show no improvement in outcomes

In either case, the spread team should gather direct feedback from adopters to refine the spread plan.

The spread team should ask the following questions to assist in the review:

- Are managers at the local level supporting the work?

- Do adopters need more or different information about how to make the changes?

- Do the communication methods to assist adopters in taking action need to be improved? Should methods be added to the communication plan?

- Do adopters have sufficient time to test and implement the changes?

- Do adopters possess sufficient understanding of improvement methods (i.e., testing and implementation)?

- Is technical support sufficient?

- Are there transition issues preventing adopters from moving to action?

4 and 5. Feedback and Maintaining the Gains. As the rate of adoption of the ideas increases and performance of the system improves, the spread team needs to ensure that structures are in place to maintain the gains achieved. Middle managers will have ownership of the new system and ultimate responsibility for feedback to adopters on performance. The spread team, therefore, should involve middle managers in each phase of its spread strategy. The spread team should assist middle managers on the appropriate measurement and audits to establish a feedback system at the local level.

Summary

This chapter describes a framework to develop and execute a spread strategy—a framework developed from theory and experience and refined over time. The framework is organized around three connected phases: (1) determining organizational readiness for spread, (2) developing an initial spread plan, and (3) executing and refining the spread plan. These phases are also the basis for the Spread Work Plan and Time Line (see Appendix 1, pages 22–24).

References

1. Rogers E.: *Diffusion of Innovations,* 4th ed. New York City: The Free Press, 1995.
2. Bandura A.: *Social Foundations of Thought and Action.* Englewood Cliffs, NJ: Prentice Hall, 1986.
3. Kotler P., Roberto E.: *Social Marketing: Strategies for Changing Public Behavior.* New York City: The Free Press, 1989.
4. Prochaska J., Norcross J., DiClemente C.: *Changing for Good.* New York City: William Morrow & Co., 1994.
5. Meteer J., et al.: Global improvement initiatives. *Multinational Business Review* 12:111–120, Spring 2004.
6. Spergel L.: Fistula First: The National Vascular Access Improvement Initiative. *Renal Physicians Association (RPA) News,* Mar. 2005, pp. 5–8.
7. Massoud M.R., et al.: *A Framework for Spread: From Local Improvement to System-Wide Change.* IHI Innovation Series white paper. Cambridge, MA: Institute for Healthcare Improvement, 2006. http://www.ihi.org/IHI/Results/WhitePapers/AFrameworkforSpreadWhitePaper.htm (accessed Jul. 3, 2007).
8. Nolan K., et al.: Using a framework for spread: The case of patient access in the Veterans Health Administration. *Jt Comm J Qual Saf* 31:339–347, Jun. 2005.
9. Schall M.W., et al.: Improving patient access to the Veterans Health Administration's primary care and specialty clinics. *Jt Comm J Qual Saf* 30:415–423, Aug. 2004.
10. Nolan K., Nielsen G., Schall M.: Developing strategies to spread improvement. In *From Front Office to Front Line: Essential Issues for Health Care Leaders.* Oakbrook Terrace, IL: Joint Commissions Resources, 2005, pp. 145–178.
11. Sirkin, H., Keenan P., Jackson A.: The hard side of change management. *Harv Bus Rev* 83:108–118, 158, Oct. 2005.
12. Galbraith J.: *Designing Organizations: An Executive Guide to Strategy, Structure, and Process.* San Francisco: Jossey-Bass, 2002.
13. Langley G.J., et al.: *The Improvement Guide: A Practical Approach to Enhancing Organizational Performance.* San Francisco: Jossey-Bass, 1996.
14. Hirschhorn L.: Campaigning for change. *Harv Bus Rev* 80:98–104, Jul. 2002.
15. Attewell P.: Technology diffusion and organizational learning. *Organization Science* 3:1–18, Feb. 1992.
16. Fraser S.: *Accelerating the Spread of Good Practice.* West Sussex, U.K.: Kingsham Press, 2002.
17. Avorn J., Soumerai S.: Improving drug therapy decisions through educational outreach. *N Engl J Med* 308:1457–1463, Jun. 16, 1983.
18. Szulanski G., Winter S.: Getting it right the second time. *Harv Bus Rev* 80:62–69, Jan. 2002.
19. Wegner E., McDermott R., Snyder W.: *Cultivating Communities of Practice.* Boston: Harvard Business School Press, 2002.

20. Katz E. The two-step flow of communication: An up-to-date report on hypothesis. *Public Opinion Quarterly* 21:61–78, Spring 1957.
21. Lomas J., et al.: Opinion leaders vs audit and feedback to implement practice guidelines: Delivery after previous cesarean section. *JAMA* 265:2202–2207, May 1, 1991.
22. Soumerai S.B., et al.: Effect of local medical opinion leaders on quality care for acute myocardial infarction: A randomized controlled trial. *JAMA* 279:1358–1363, May 6, 1998.
23. Gladwell M.: *The Tipping Point.* Boston: Little, Brown and Company, 2000.
24. Brown J., Duguid P.: *The Social Life of Foundation.* Boston: Harvard Business School Press, 2000.
25. Dixon N.M.: *Common Knowledge: How Companies Thrive by Sharing What They Know.* Boston: Harvard Business School Press, 2000
26. Cool K., Dierickx I., Szulanski G.: Diffusion of innovations within organizations: Electronic switching in the Bell System, 1971–1982. *Organization Science* 8:543–559, Sep./Oct. 1997.
27. Bass F.: A new product growth model for consumer durables. *Management Science* 13:215–227, Jan. 1969.
28. Brown J., Duguid P.: How to capture knowledge without killing it. *Harv Bus Rev* 78: 73–80, May–Jun. 2000.

Appendix 1-1.
SPREAD WORK PLAN AND TIME LINE

Develop and Execute a Spread Strategy

Determining Organizational Readiness → Developing an Initial Spread Plan → Executing and Refining the Spread Plan

Spread Activity	What We Will Do…	Start Date	Responsible Person
Phase 1. Determing Organizational Readiness			
Select a topic			
Ensure executive sponsorship			
Assign a day-to-day manager			
Form a spread team			
Identify successful sites			
Develop the case			
Describe the ideas			

Appendix 1-1. (continued)
SPREAD WORK PLAN AND TIME LINE

Spread Activity	What We Will Do…	Start Date	Responsible Person
Phase 2. Developing an Initial Spread Plan			
Develop an Aim			
Identify what will be spread			
State the level of performance			
Identify the target population			
Specify the time frame			
Describe how the structure of the organization can be leveraged			
Communication			
Identify the target audience(s) and "messages" for each			
List the ways that members typically exchange information			
Specify communication methods or channels for awareness			

Appendix 1-1. (continued)
SPREAD WORK PLAN AND TIME LINE

Spread Activity	What We Will Do...	Start Date	Responsible Person
Specify communication methods for knowledge transfer to move adopters to action			
Describe how you will use key messengers or mentors (who know the improvements)			
Measurement			
Develop methods to collect the data in your aim statement			
Develop methods to track rate of adoption of the interventions			
Phase 3. Executing and Refining the Spread Plan			
Identify ways to provide feedback to adopters			
Identify ways to gather information to allow for adjustment of the spread plan			
Identify "transition issues," e.g., barriers to implementation and ways to overcome them			

Chapter 2
Eliminating Facility-Acquired Pressure Ulcers at Ascension Health

Wanda Gibbons, R.N., M.H.A.
Helana T. Shanks, R.N.
Pam Kleinhelter, R.N., M.S.N.
Polly Jones, L.C.S.W.

Background and Overview

Ascension Health (http://www.ascensionhealth.org) is the largest Catholic and not-for-profit system in the United States. More than 101,000 associates and 25,000 physicians (including approximately 1,500 employed physicians) provide care to more than 660,000 hospitalized patients a year in 65 hospitals throughout 20 states and the District of Columbia.

In 2004, Ascension Health established a goal of zero preventable injuries and deaths within all facilities by July 2008. Nine alpha sites were established to define best practices to eliminate potentially preventable complications occurring in its health care facilities.[1] These initiatives have been incorporated into eight priorities for action (Table 2-1, page 26). St. Vincent's Medical Center, as an alpha site, was charged with defining best practices to eliminate facility-acquired pressure ulcers—best practices that could then be spread throughout Ascension Health. This initiative was a strategic priority for both Ascension Health and St. Vincent's Medical Center, as reflected in St. Vincent's goals, reward systems, and measurements, and was implemented through an organizational transformational change process.

Pressure ulcers are areas of localized tissue destruction caused by the compression of soft tissue over a bony prominence and an external surface for a prolonged period of time. Pressure ulcers, staged from I through IV to classify the degree of damage observed,[2] can develop within 24 hours of skin injury or appear as late as 5 days post-injury.[3]

Hundreds of articles have been written regarding the prevention and treatment of pressure ulcers. Several groups, including the Wound Ostomy and Continence Nurses (WOCN) Society and the National Pressure Ulcer Advisory Panel, have reviewed the literature regarding etiology, risk factors, prevention, and treatment of pressure ulcers. Best practice guidelines have been published on the basis of their expert reviews.[2,4] The WOCN Society estimates that more than one million persons in the United States develop pressure ulcers each year.[5] The incidence of pressure ulcers has been estimated to range from 0.4% to 38% of patients in acute care settings, with 48% to 53% of these pressure ulcers occurring while the patient is hospitalized.[4] The 2006 International Pressure Ulcer Prevalence Study, sponsored by Hill-Rom, reported a pressure ulcer prevalence of 13.8% and a hospital-acquired pressure ulcer prevalence of

Table 2-1.
ASCENSION HEALTH PRIORITIES FOR ACTION

Preventable Mortality

Adverse Drug Events

Joint Commission National Patient Safety Goals and Core Measures

Nosocomial Infections

Perioperative Complications

Falls

Pressure Ulcers

Perinatal Safety

6.3%.[6] For the purposes of its initiative, St. Vincent's Medical Center defined a facility-acquired pressure ulcer as any pressure ulcer that was not documented within 24 hours of admission.

The mean cost per hospital admission for patients who develop a pressure ulcer has been reported to be $37,288,[7] which translates into a cost of $2.2 to $3.6 billion each year in acute care settings.[8] However, the financial cost paints only a partial picture of the effects of pressure ulcers. The human cost can be pain, debilitation, and even death.

Aim of the Spread Initiative

The aim of the spread initiative was the elimination of facility-acquired pressure ulcers throughout Ascension Health. St. Vincent's Medical Center served as the alpha site to develop a comprehensive program for spread. The principal ideas spread were head-to-toe skin assessments, risk assessments every shift, and implementation of the SKIN bundle (see page 27) for patients at risk. The development of this program ensured that all Ascension Health facilities would have the tools necessary to reach the outcome-oriented goal of zero preventable facility-acquired pressure ulcers. The target population included all patients admitted to Ascension Health facilities. A time line for alpha site development and implementation was developed to ensure full implementation at the alpha site by December 2005 and systemwide by 2007.

St. Vincent's Medical Center: The Alpha Site Initiative

A faith-based, mission-driven health care provider, St. Vincent's Medical Center is a 528-bed licensed facility and the largest hospital provider of adult inpatient services in northeast Florida, with an 18% market share. This translates into 26,600 admissions, 2,200 deliveries, and 64,000 emergency department (ED) visits annually.

St. Vincent's Medical Center volunteered, and was selected, to develop the process for the prevention of pressure ulcers. Our organization had focused on reducing pressure ulcer prevalence and incidence in 2000–2002, when we observed increasing costs for specialty-bed rentals associated with the treatment of pressure ulcers. On the basis of this recent experience and strong support from the nursing staff, St. Vincent's believed that the alpha initiative would be a natural fit for our organization. In addition, we considered pressure ulcer prevention an opportunity for our nurses to drive a process to positively affect patient outcomes and increase our pride in professional nursing practice.

Because Ascension Health comprises facilities offering services ranging from acute care to long term care, we described the initiative as "facility" rather than "hospital" focused. We planned to disseminate the results and benefits of the initiative throughout Ascension Health.

The initiative for the prevention of facility-acquired pressure ulcers, a strategic priority for St. Vincent's Medical Center, was clearly reflected in the goals, reward systems, and measurements. More importantly, the organization's board of directors had designated it as one of a small set of priorities. Individual performance goals for the chief executive officer, chief operating officer, chief nursing officer (CNO), nursing directors, and nurse managers were aligned with the pressure ulcer prevention effort. Because the prevention of pressure ulcers is primarily a nursing-driven process, the CNO [W.G.] assumed executive sponsorship of the initiative.

As shown in the time line for the pressure ulcer initiative (Table 2, right), the leadership team was established in February 2004. The team was composed of the CNO, a nurse manager [P.K.], educators [including H.S.], a pharmacist, a dietitian, two staff nurses, two WOCN Society–registered nurses (RNs), a nurse in performance improvement, and a long term care nursing educator. The nurse manager and clinical educator had day-to-day responsibility for keeping the initiative moving, with support from the CNO and the entire nursing leadership team.

After forming the team, the next step was to review the current policies and procedures and conduct a literature review of best practices, in preparation for an "expert" meeting held in June 2004. Representatives from the Institute for Healthcare Improvement and Ascension Health, as well as WOCN Society experts from across the United States, met with the team to create a blueprint for the change package, which included promising intervention ideas, a time line, and key concepts. For example, the facility already used a risk assessment tool, the Braden Scale for Predicting Pressure Sore Risk,[9] in daily assessments, and the expert meeting confirmed the need to continue to use this evidence-based tool.

After the expert meeting, we developed the SKIN bundle in July 2004 as a synergistic group of interventions to enable us to guide the initiative. This bundle addressed interventions related to the **S**urfaces, or mattresses and cushions on which the patients lay or sit, the need to **K**eep the patients turning or moving, the need to manage **I**ncontinence, and the importance of **N**utrition and hydration. Henceforth, we referred to the alpha initiative leadership as the SKIN team.

With the team in place, we were ready to go "live" with the first three nursing units in August 2004.

Preparation for the Alpha Site Initiative

Culture Modification
Before the start of the pressure ulcer prevention program, the incidence of pressure ulcers at St. Vincent's was lower than national norms and Ascension averages. Specifically, the facility-acquired pressure ulcer prevalence was 5.7%,

Table 2-2. PRESSURE ULCER PREVENTION PROGRAM TIME LINE*

February 2004   Formation of pressure ulcer team
May 2004   Review of literature   Prevalence study
June 2004   Expert meeting
July 2004   Bundle developed
August 2004   First 3 units "go live"
September 2004   Operations management meetings started
October 2004   Further rollout to units   Test surfaces in OR/ED   Change in products
November 2004   All units completed   Replaced 162 surfaces or mattresses
December 2004   Continuation of weekly skin operations meetings   Prevalence study

*The program was rolled out to all units in December 2004; OR, operating room; ED, emergency department. Used with permission.

compared with the Ascension Health average of 7.6% and a national average of 7.7% in the 2004 Hill-Rom International Pressure Ulcer Prevalence Survey.[10] However, to reach the target—the elimination of facility-acquired pressure ulcers—we determined that several aspects of the organizational culture needed modification. Some staff believed that pressure ulcers were unavoidable in complex, critically ill patients—that maintaining heart and lung functions overshadowed the need for skin care and pressure ulcer prevention. We could not be satisfied with this traditional view. We changed the expectation from "critically ill patients will leave the organization alive" to "critically ill patients will leave the organization alive and without pressure ulcers." The culture changes were incorporated during handoff communications, in which the caregivers began to consistently include the status of patients' skin.

Not only did we raise the bar on our expectations of what we considered acceptable with regard to pressure ulcers, we also made clear to the staff that this initiative would endure as the start of a ground-breaking change in patient care. A significant impetus to the culture change was the empowerment of the staff. From the first in-service and throughout the initiative, caregivers at the bedside influenced the process. Their knowledge and experience were valued, and their pride was enhanced as they improved patient outcomes and built a national model for best practice. On the basis of the feedback of bedside caregivers in the first pilot unit, St. Vincent's changed compression stockings, adopting a product less likely to contribute to breakdowns on the dorsum of the foot.

Nursing directors, nurse managers, clinical resource coordinators, and unit champions attended weekly SKIN operations meetings—debriefings with the nursing leadership—where pressure ulcer incidence was reviewed. Led by a nursing director, SKIN operations meetings provided a forum in which knowledge and experience were shared and techniques for promoting staff accountability were discussed.

Internal Research/Rationale for Pilot Units at St. Vincent's Medical Center

Before we educated staff and implemented the SKIN bundle, we reviewed charts of 30 patients who had developed pressure ulcers in the previous six months. The review revealed an increased risk for patients with one or more co-morbidities among four diagnoses: congestive heart failure, sepsis, respiratory failure, and renal failure. Of the 30 patients, 22 had a history of cardiovascular disease. Partly on the basis of these findings, we chose the following units as the pilot units:

- The 8-bed open heart recovery unit
- The 28-bed cardiovascular progressive care unit
- The 14-bed coronary care unit

Once the data were communicated to these units, the caregiver staff were eager to initiate the pilot and reduce the rate of facility-acquired pressure ulcers. In fact, one of the initially vocal and reluctant staff members became the strongest advocate and cheerleader for the program once she reviewed the data and observed the change in patient outcomes with the SKIN bundle.

According to chart reviews, for 87% of the time, a nutritional consult had been ordered for patients with pressure ulcers, but the nutritional recommendations were followed only 35% of the time. We therefore instituted an immediate practice change. Dietitians had previously written their recommendations in the multidisciplinary progress notes, where they could be lost in the shuffle of paperwork, so St. Vincent's revised its process and created medical staff–approved standing orders for dietitians. Although these specific standing orders are not required as part of the nutrition portion of the bundle throughout Ascension Health, they were shared with all Ascension Health facilities as one method to ensure physician support and document physician orders for nutrition and hydration supplementation.

Once we completed the chart review and identified the pilot units, we began implementation and measurement of the program. We educated the staff, refined implementation of the program, and recorded and reported the results, as described in the following section.

Spread Within St. Vincent's Medical Center

The education plan for the pressure ulcer prevention initiative included the following components:

- Identification of core responsibilities for each member of the team responsible for pressure ulcer prevention

- Development of educational offerings for each audience—for example, licensed and unlicensed clinical staff, unit champions/experts, and the executive team
- Development of the SKIN bundle
- Teaching that skin is an organ system
- Presentation of the initiative as a nursing-driven process, emphasizing pride of practice.

The clinical components of staff education included the etiology and risk factors that predispose patients to develop pressure ulcers and interventions to minimize risk. Nurses' knowledge of skin assessment using the Braden scale, staging of pressure ulcers using the National Pressure Ulcer Advisory Panel guidelines,[3] and selection of appropriate surfaces were reinforced. We taught the staff to develop and implement an individualized plan of skin care and to accurately document pertinent data. Licensed and unlicensed clinical staff attended the same educational, orientation, and unit educational programs, which included skin assessment during patient care, such as bathing and turning.

A brief presentation to all clinical staff introduced the SKIN bundle and included the elements. The educators also provided the background, structure, rationale, and results anticipated with implementation of the SKIN bundle. Education began with the three pilot units, *followed by a staggered rollout of the initiative to all nursing units during a four-month period.* Units were selected for the rollout on the basis of their facility-acquired pressure ulcer rate as well as leadership and staff support for the initiative. When possible, units with similar patient populations (for example, surgical, cardiovascular) were rolled out together. Initial data from the pilot units were promising (Figure 2-1, below).

Figure 2-1.
PILOT UNITS: FACILITY-ACQUIRED PRESSURE ULCER RATE, AUGUST 2004–JUNE 2005

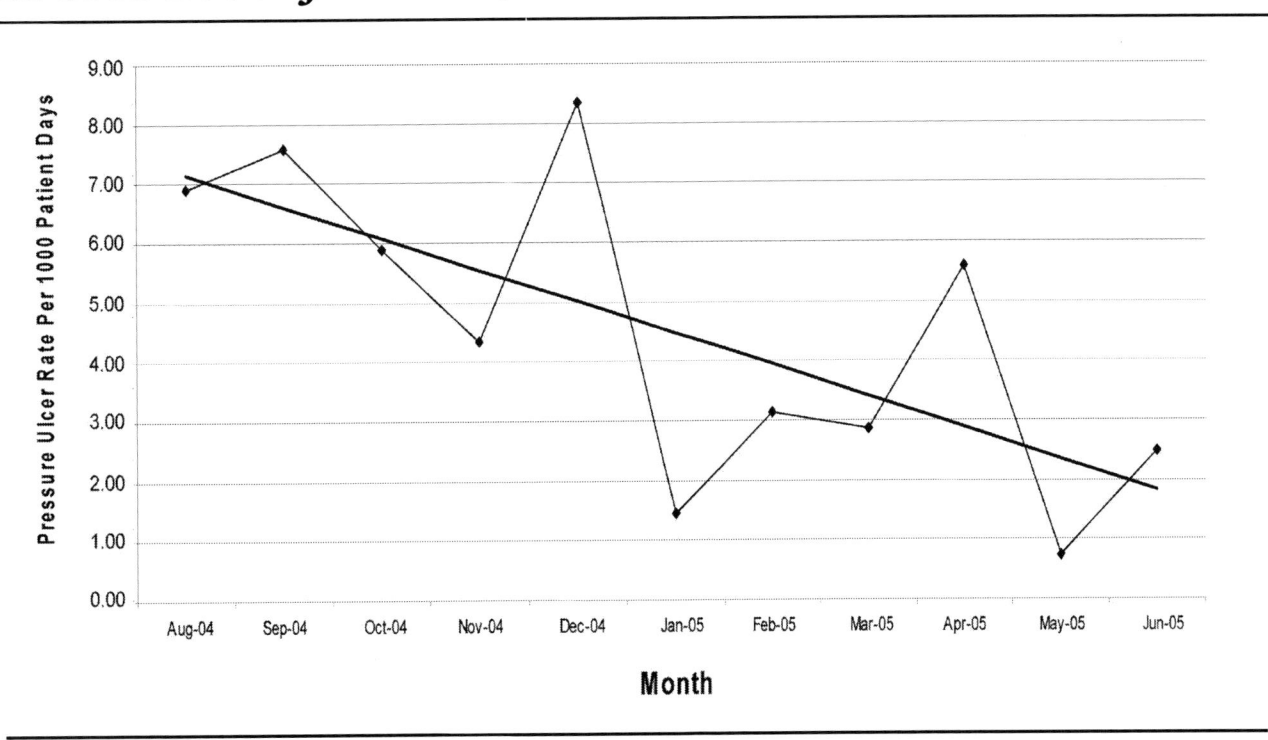

The reduction in facility-acquired pressure ulcer rate by month per 1,000 patient days on three pilot units, August 2004–June 2005, is shown. Used with permission.

All units adopted and implemented the SKIN bundle by the end of 2004. Through our weekly SKIN operations team meetings, we monitored each unit's progress in reducing facility-acquired pressure ulcers. We observed unit-to-unit variation in bundle compliance for at least six months as a consistent philosophy of skin assessment, and interventions became the culture on each unit. The review of each pressure ulcer to identify unit-level actions to prevent a similar future facility-acquired pressure ulcer was essential to the ongoing, sustained decrease in pressure ulcers. We continued to learn and change processes following full implementation of the bundle. Additional education in the rollout included bedside teaching of the application of all elements of the SKIN bundle, newsletters highlighting individual components of the bundle, self-study modules related to assessment and prevention of pressure ulcers, placement of a poster (Figure 2-2, right) in prominent areas on the individual nursing units, and pocket reference cards of the Braden scale and staging. For all patients with a Braden score of ≤ 18, which indicates increased risk of developing a pressure ulcer, a reminder of the SKIN bundle was placed on their nursing documentation clipboards (Figure 2-3, page 31).

Routine ongoing education efforts in the pressure ulcer prevention initiative included education of new staff in orientation and continuing education for all licensed and unlicensed staff regarding updates or changes in process. Education was also provided to all staff through participation in quarterly prevalence study teams as well as during shift-to-shift reports. We assessed educational needs versus compliance issues when we identified a decline in performance indicators. For unexpected spikes in incidence in which the SKIN bundle was documented, we conducted chart reviews in an effort to isolate and address causative factors. Factors not addressed in the SKIN bundle, such as poor tissue perfusion, were addressed through continued literature searches, discussion, and planning.

Implementation Refinements
After the pressure ulcer prevention program was introduced to the units, each unit's leadership was expected to monitor and report compliance with the SKIN bundle and related issues in weekly SKIN operations meetings. Also every week, each unit reviewed charts of all high-risk patients for compliance with the bundle and provided a report on a specially developed tool (Figure 2-4, page 32). This review proved to be very beneficial to the process because any issues with products or processes were brought forward and

Figure 2-2.
POSTER FOR SKIN INITIATIVE

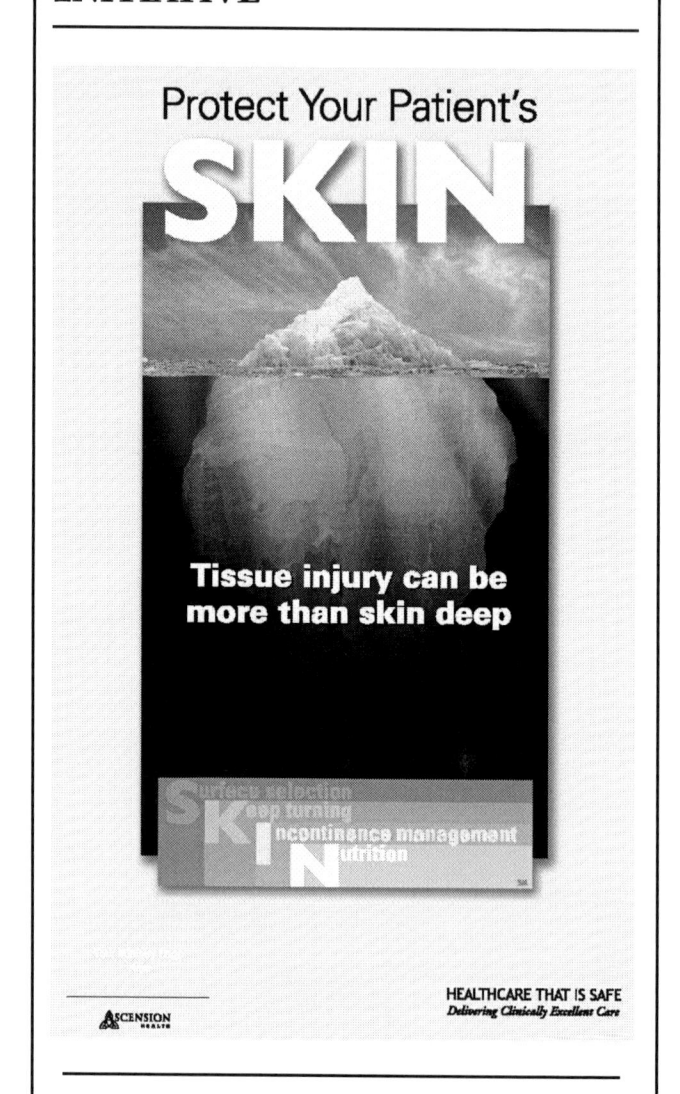

This poster was placed in prominent areas on the individual nursing units at St. Vincent's Medical Center. Used with permission.

Figure 2-3.
SKIN RISK ALERT REMINDER TO NURSES

SKIN RISK ALERT
SKIN BUNDLE INTERVENTIONS IN EFFECT!

SURFACE:
- Be sure patient is on correct type of mattress.
- Do not use multiple layers of linens under patient.
- Keep linens free of wrinkles.
- Be sure patient is not lying on tubing, telephones or call bells.

KEEP TURNING:
- Reposition patient at least every two hours when in bed.
- "Self" is not acceptable for documenting repositioning.
- Document the actual position the patient is observed in.
- Shift patient's weight at least every hour if up in chair.
- Use a chair pad when patient up in a chair.

INCONTINENCE:
- Offer toileting assistance every two hours.
- If incontinent, give perineal care every two hours and as needed for stool incontinence.
- Apply a moisture barrier after incontinence care.
- If not incontinent, apply moisture barrier every 8 hours.
- Avoid diapers unless needed for containing excessive amounts of stool, patient is ambulatory and incontinent or saturates linens with most urinary incontinence episodes or patient requests diaper.

NUTRITION:
- If patient has a nutritional deficit or is high risk for a nutritional deficit, order a nutrition consult. Look at what the patient has been taking in for nutrition and also look at albumin levels.
- Consider recent weight loss as well.
- Consider hydration status.
- Carry out nutrition orders and record supplement and meal intake.

Assess skin every eight hours. Document breakdown description on Skin Flow Sheet daily.

Document all of your interventions.

Not a permanent part of the medical record

The S (surface), K (keep turning), I (incontinence management), and N (nutrition) risk reminder was placed on nursing clipboards for patients at risk of pressure ulcers. Used with permission.

Figure 2-4.
SKIN Bundle Compliance Tool

Pt identifier										
Braden score < 18										
LOS > 48 hours										
S Surface type										
K Turning documented q 2										
K Heels off bed documented										
I Incontinence care documented										
N Nutritionally at risk										
N Nutritional consult completed										
N Nutritional orders written										
N Nutritional orders carried out										
Comments										

The pressure ulcer prevention monitoring tool was developed for compliance with documentation of the S (surface), K (keep turning), I (incontinence management), and N (nutrition) bundle. LOS, length of stay. Used with permission.

investigated weekly. For example, on the basis of the work of the SKIN operations meetings, we adopted a fecal incontinence collection system and adult diapers and disposable underpads that contained less plastic. The operating room (OR) and ED trialed the use of different surfaces for patients at increased risk of developing pressure ulcers. The OR adopted special surfaces for patients whose OR times were expected to be greater than or equal to three hours. Similarly, the ED attempted to place patients on special surfaces when long ED waits were expected.

Results

Before beginning the alpha site work, St. Vincent's monitored pressure ulcers per 1,000 discharges, reported data for facility- and community-acquired pressure ulcers, and maintained a database with pertinent data on all pressure ulcers. As we progressed with the alpha initiative, we found that these metrics did not provide robust data that met the goal of timely, easily accessible, and meaningful data at both the organization and unit level. Specifically, we were unable to track a pressure ulcer rate at the unit level because a patient may develop a pressure ulcer in one unit but be discharged from another unit. In addition, the facility-wide discharge metric was reported on a monthly basis. Hence, we modified the metric to the number of pressure ulcers per 1,000 *patient days*, with the pressure ulcer allocated to the unit on which it was initially observed. St. Vincent's calculates facility-acquired pressure ulcer ratios on weekly, monthly, and quarterly bases. We also conduct a quarterly prevalence survey and an annual incidence survey to validate the ongoing measures.

A downward trend of pressure ulcer incidence at St. Vincent's was evident (Figure 2-5, page 34), decreasing from > 2% to < 1% from January 2004 through March 2007. The difference in the number of facility-acquired pressure ulcers per 1,000 patient days between January 2004 to April 2005 and May 2005 to March 2007 was statistically significant ($p < .05$).

More importantly, no new Stage IV facility-acquired pressure ulcers occurred between August 2004 and May 2007 (the most recent month for which data were available).

Only two facility-acquired Stage III pressure ulcers occurred during this 33-month period. One of the staff's initial frustrations was that the number of pressure ulcers did not quickly reduce to and sustain at zero. In fact, following the initial staff education, the number of reported facility-acquired pressure ulcers temporarily increased. Anecdotal evidence suggested that the staff were assessing skin regularly and identifying ulcers earlier in the skin breakdown process, factors that could increase reported incidence. Despite the initial increase in incidence, the staff thought the pressure ulcers were smaller and healing faster. Through the weekly SKIN operations meetings and use of the SKIN process tool, we knew that 100% of the at-risk patients were being evaluated for appropriate interventions, including nutrition orders. Although implementation of the SKIN bundle occurred during the time period of August–December 2004, full adoption of the bundle and culture change continued through mid-2005. At approximately five to six months following housewide implementation, organizational results were significantly improved, reflecting the staff's complete buy-in on the importance of evaluating skin as an organ system and their consistent changes in day-to-day clinical practice.

Following the SKIN bundle implementation at St. Vincent's, we continued to monitor all facility-acquired pressure ulcers, conduct quarterly prevalence studies, and identify other opportunities to reduce and eliminate facility-acquired pressure ulcers. One recent prevalence study, conducted in November 2006, demonstrated a facility-acquired prevalence rate of 0.86%. Local (hospital) experts expressed concern about fragile skin in the elderly and the impact of hypoperfusion in complex medical and surgical patients. We began to develop a skin fragility assessment tool, evaluate hypoperfusion and its impact on the prevalence of pressure ulcers, and pay special attention to skin pigmentation. Skin failure is an area of further study.

Spread to the Other Ascension Health Facilities

The alpha site work and SKIN bundle were presented to nursing colleagues from all 67 Ascension Health acute care facilities at the rapid-design-format Pressure Ulcer Summit in St. Louis May 31 to June 1, 2005. High-level, preliminary

Figure 2-5.
ST. VINCENT'S MEDICAL CENTER FACILITY-ACQUIRED PRESSURE ULCER RATE BY MONTH, JANUARY 2004–MARCH 2007

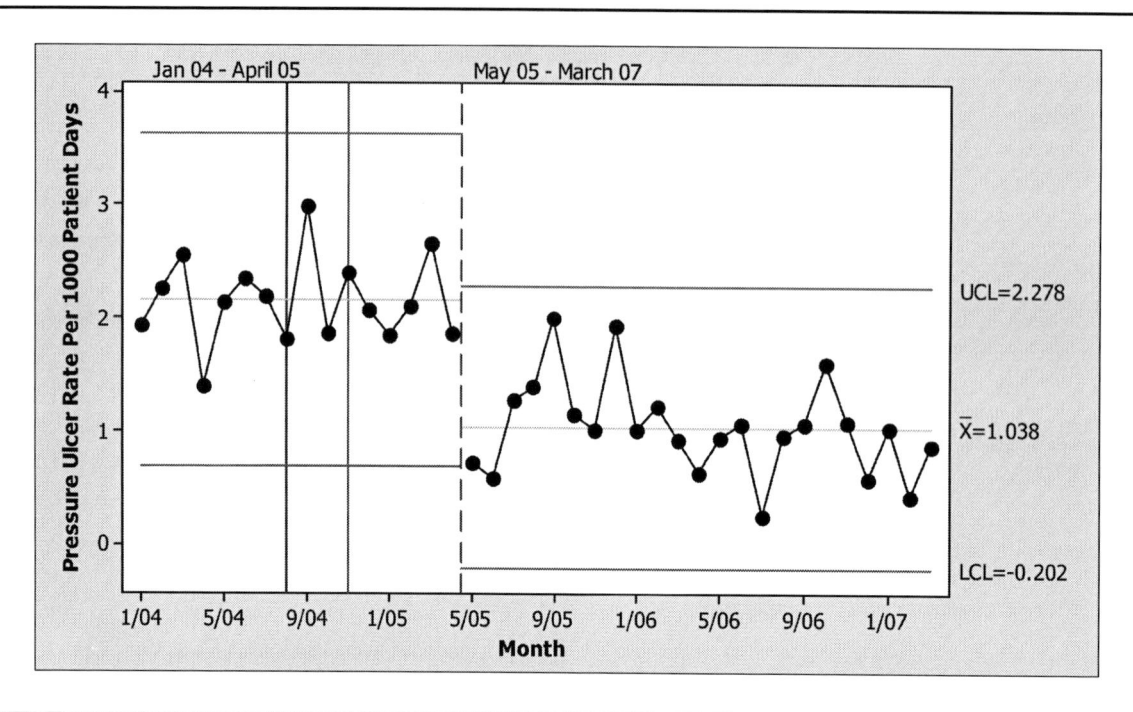

The reduction in facility-acquired pressure ulcer rate by month per 1,000 patient days, January 2004–March 2007, St. Vincent's Medical Center, is shown. Implementation occurred between August 2004 and December 2004, as indicated by the vertical lines. UCL, upper control limit; LCL, lower control limit. Used with permission.

information and early results from the pressure ulcer initiative at St. Vincent's had been shared with various Ascension audiences, including the 12-member CNO advisory council and 12-member clinical excellence team (which is empowered to act on behalf of the clinical leaders to provide overall clinical direction).

On the basis of the early success at St. Vincent's, these groups supported and sponsored the Pressure Ulcer Summit to provide the SKIN bundle to all Ascension facilities and determine the optimal methodology for spread. A couple other facilities had also begun implementation of the SKIN bundle. These early adopters purchased new surfaces or beds and experienced similar improvement in reduction of facility-acquired pressure ulcers as the alpha site.

Under the leadership of the facility CNOs, each facility was invited to send five nurses to the 2005 summit. Attendees included CNOs, clinical educators, wound experts, front-line nurse managers, and clinical staff nurses. The summit's specific goals were as follows:

- Raise awareness about the success at St. Vincent's so other facilities would make the decision to adopt the changes.

- Create and adopt the preferred practice(s) to eliminate facility-acquired pressure ulcers and define best practice for the care of all pressure ulcers.

- Create a project time line.

- Define measurement criteria, goals, and definitions.

We described St. Vincent's model and experiences with pressure ulcer prevention, and colleagues from the other facilities had an opportunity to share their best practices and enhance the program.

Summit participants voiced unanimous support for a standardized pressure ulcer assessment, prevention, and treatment program throughout Ascension Health. All acute care facilities agreed to a single model of care using the SKIN bundle and common measures of quality and performance—and committed to implementing the SKIN bundle by January 1, 2006.

Subsequent meetings were held to address aspects of the SKIN bundle for pediatric and long term care populations. The final recommendations were distributed to all Ascension Health facilities with a tool kit (documentation of best practices, implementation techniques, and tools for use in changing practices) in November 2005. The tool kit also included Ascension Health–branded materials for use in the pressure ulcer prevention journey at each facility, as shown in Figure 2-6 (right).

The Ascension Health CNO group assumed accountability for the successful spread and implementation of the pressure ulcer initiative. The CNO advisory council meets monthly to provide strategic direction and thought leadership on major system-related topic areas that are deemed to affect quality, safety, staffing and operational performance, nursing leadership, product evaluation/acquisition, and patient care delivery. Each member of this group then follows up with a "pod"—a group of six to eight other CNOs within Ascension Health. Through this shared governance decision-making process, Ascension Health is able to vet major system issues across the entire CNO leadership for consensus building and action.

Affinity groups and monthly calls were also established to connect associates from the various health facilities on the topic of pressure ulcers. The monthly calls were attended by at least one representative from each Ascension Health facility. The agendas for the affinity calls cover a variety of topics, from clinical issues to change management and recent research findings.

Figure 2-6.
EXAMPLES OF ASCENSION HEALTH–BRANDED MATERIALS FOR SKIN INITIATIVES

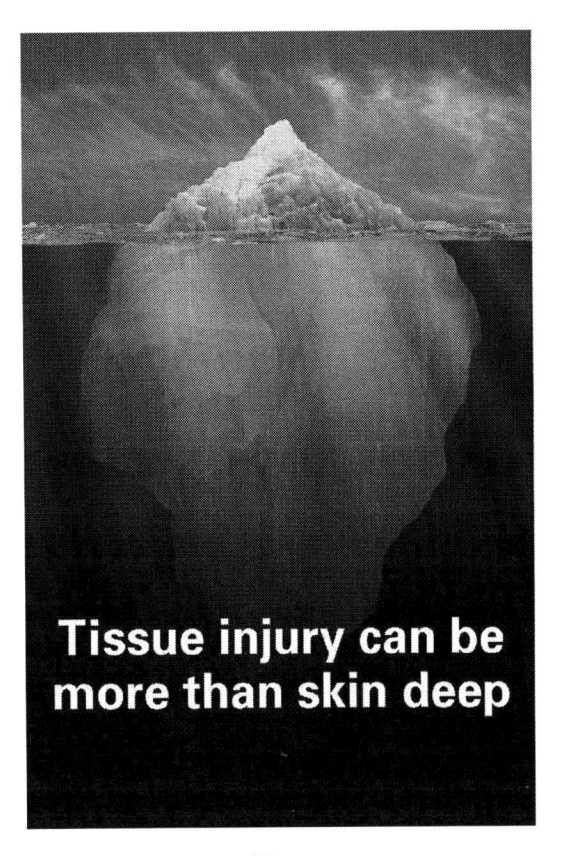

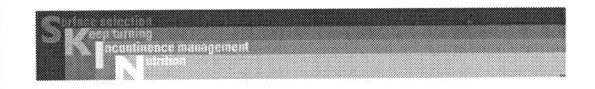

Examples of Ascension Health–branded materials for S (surface), K (keep turning), I (incontinence), and N (nutrition) initiatives are shown. Used with permission.

Key elements of the successful spread of the initiative are summarized in Table 2-3 (below). The alpha site's work was critical in the development of a comprehensive program that could then be shared with the other Ascension Health facilities. Leadership of local health facilities ministries, specifically CNO support, enabled the pressure ulcer initiative to spread to all facilities. Availability of ongoing support such as listserves, affinity groups, and conference calls, as well as material from the tool kit, provided additional impetus for spread. Finally, regular reports on outcome measures helped monitor the progress in the pressure ulcer initiative.

As agreed at the 2005 Pressure Ulcer Summit, every Ascension Health hospital has adopted the standardized assessment, prevention, and treatment program. Both St. Vincent's and the early adopters provided consultation to other facilities as they began the implementation process during the six months following the summit. During this period of implementation, monthly calls were held, during which participants could share issues related to implementation and receive continuing education to strengthen the work done by the alpha site. The listserve enabled staff in Ascension Health facilities to network with their colleagues and receive help with implementation and other questions. Each CNO and his or her leadership team determined the optimal method of spread within their facility—whether it was a methodical, linear, unit-by-unit spread or a concurrent, housewide "go-live" process. By the end of the first quarter of 2006, all Ascension Health acute care facilities had fully implemented the SKIN bundle. By the second quarter of 2007, more than 50% of the bed fleet was upgraded to pressure redistribution surfaces.

To monitor ongoing progress toward the system goal of zero preventable facility-acquired pressure ulcers, each facility within Ascension Health was asked to submit the number of facility-acquired pressure ulcers identified each month into a system database. Figure 2-7 (page 37) demonstrates the downward trend in the rate of pressure ulcers per 1,000 patient days. The system experienced a 36% reduction in the first 15 months of implementation of the recommendations tested at the alpha site. Figure 2-8 (page 38) compares the facility-acquired pressure ulcer prevalence as reported in the 2005 and 2007 Hill-Rom International Prevalence Studies. Ascension Health experienced a 43.4% reduction in facility-acquired pressure ulcer prevalence from 2005 to 2007.

A second Pressure Ulcer Summit was held May 30 to 31, 2007, in Jacksonville to celebrate the successes already achieved and to review "second-generation work." The convened nursing and other health team members from all Ascension Health facilities reviewed and adopted standardized processes to maximize the use of both processes and products to bring the rate of facility-acquired pressure ulcers even closer to zero, reduce falls resulting in injury, deliver coordinated care to bariatric patients, and reduce worker injuries due to inappropriate patient handling. Specific outcomes from the summit will be the creation of a skin failure listserve, development of a skin failure tool kit, standardization of skin failure definitions, and a plan for a large multicenter study of skin failure.

Ascension Health is also developing an innovative e-learning initiative that provides a high-tech, interactive platform to launch learning modules (including video clips and interactive scenarios) for each of its eight priorities for

Table 2-3.
KEY ELEMENTS OF SPREAD*

- Alpha site work at St. Vincent's Medical Center
- Development of SKIN bundle
- Communication of SKIN bundle at Pressure Ulcer Summit
- Consensus on single standardized plan of care and implementation of SKIN bundle
- Tool kit shared with each facility
- CNO leadership and accountability
- Strategic bed replacement plan
- Ongoing support, including listserves, affinity groups, newsletters, and conference calls
- Monthly reporting of results and communication to all facilities

*SKIN, S (surface), K (keep turning), I (incontinence management), and N (nutrition). CNO, chief nursing officer. Used with permission.

Figure 2-7.
ASCENSION HEALTH FACILITY-ACQUIRED PRESSURE ULCER RATIO BY PATIENT DAYS, JANUARY 2006–MARCH 2007

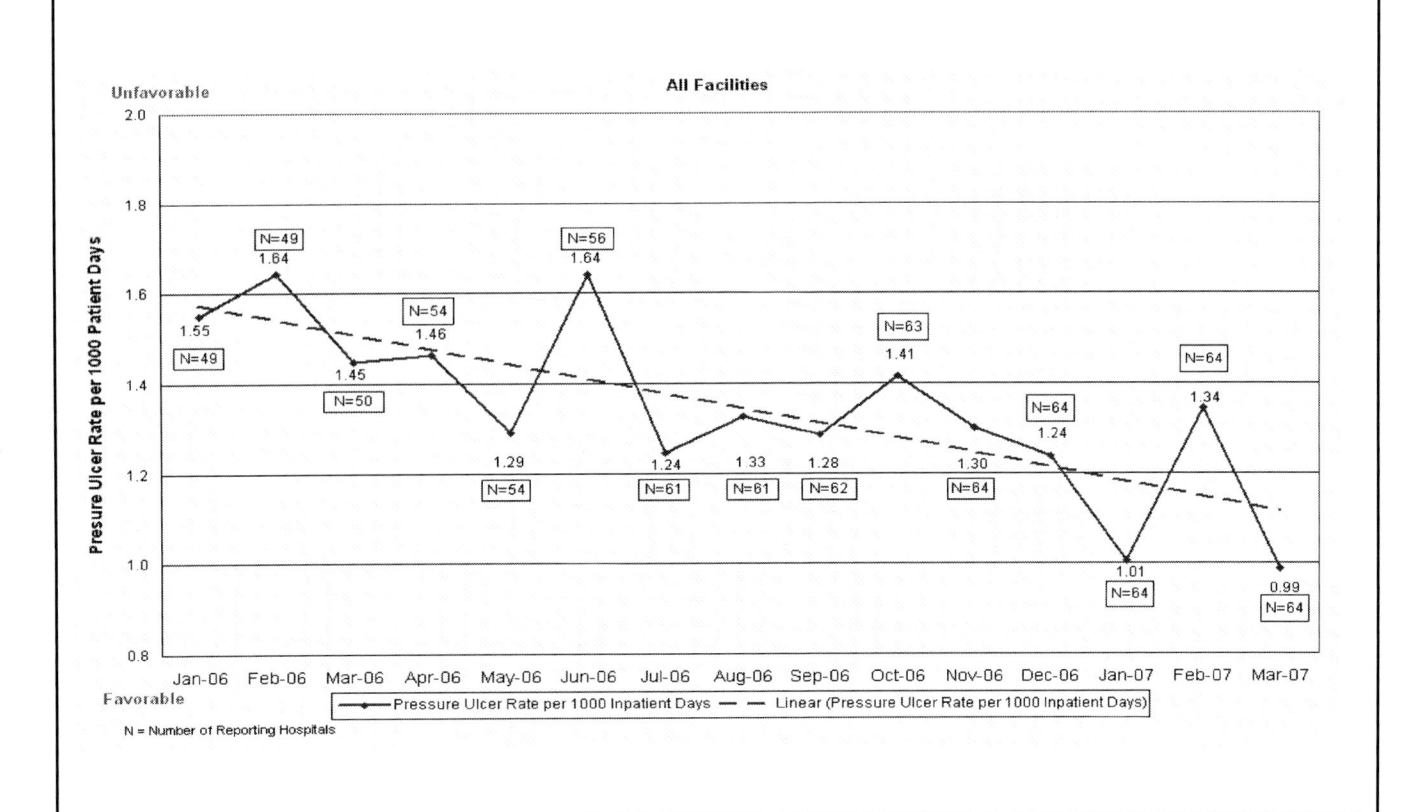

The reduction in facility-acquired pressure ulcer rate per 1,000 patient days, by reporting hospitals January 2006–January 2007, Ascension Health, is shown. Used with permission.

action, beginning with pressure ulcer prevention and maximizing the functionality of the new bed fleet delivered across the system. This proprietary pressure ulcer prevention module was successfully premiered at the summit. Feedback from summit attendees was incorporated into the final interactive e-learning modules.

Discussion

The St. Vincent's alpha site initiative in pressure ulcer prevention was based on internal and external research, which enabled St. Vincent's to identify at-risk populations, implement appropriate actions, and achieve positive, measurable, meaningful results. In addition, leadership support at all levels was essential, from the executive sponsor to the frontline supervisor, to ensure the initiative's success. In the beginning stages of an initiative such as this, the work is time and resource intensive. When the SKIN team was given uninterrupted time from other responsibilities to launch the initiative, the message was clear: There is leadership support. Although St. Vincent's incurred some incremental costs as nonproductive time for education, the facility did not add staff for this initiative.

When the rollout was complete at St. Vincent's, maintaining weekly SKIN operations meetings fostered accountability

Figure 2-8.
ASCENSION HEALTH FACILITY-ACQUIRED PRESSURE ULCER PREVALENCE, 2005 AND 2007

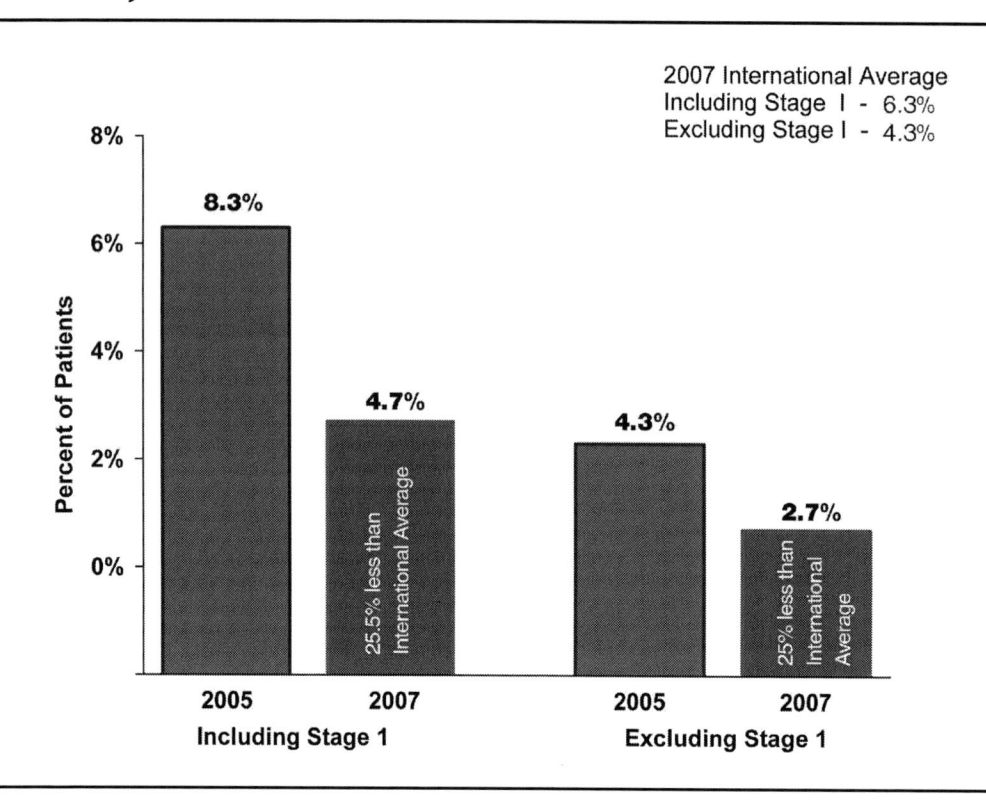

2007 International Average
Including Stage I - 6.3%
Excluding Stage I - 4.3%

Including Stage 1: 2005 = 8.3%, 2007 = 4.7% (25.5% less than International Average)
Excluding Stage 1: 2005 = 4.3%, 2007 = 2.7% (25% less than International Average)

The reduction in facility-acquired pressure ulcer prevalence in 2005 and 2007, Ascension Health, is shown. Data for the 2007 international averages are from Hill-Rom: Hill-Rom International Pressure Ulcer Prevalence Study. *Batesville, IN: Hill-Rom, 2007. Used with permission.*

from frontline supervisors, managers, and directors and continued success with the initiative. Promoting prevention of pressure ulcers as a nursing-driven process empowered nurses at all levels and encouraged staff to be proactive in seeking improved outcomes for their patients.

As we educated the staff, we learned that we could not assume that the knowledge base within disciplines was equal. Thus, we started with the basics for all licensed and unlicensed staff and then developed advanced education for the SKIN champions. We learned that educational offerings should be short, focused, and offered at multiple times and through a variety of venues, with the information presented as thoroughly to the last group as to the first.

Ongoing education should be presented whenever an opportunity arises, as when senior staff teach less experienced staff during a prevalence study.

Communication was a vital component of this initiative's success. When selecting the individuals who made up the team responsible for planning, educating, disseminating, and monitoring this process, we considered communication skills to be as important as clinical expertise. Soliciting input from staff both in the planning stages and in the rollout emphasized empowerment and pride of practice.

A key learning was that pilots do not have to be perfect. The pilot's operational processes may be affected, for example, by delays in initiating a pilot study, gathering data, or implementing treatment regimes. We made decisions, then tested and refined those decisions during the pilot. To help us stay on task, we identified target dates and used a time line. To help stay motivated, we continually celebrated our successes, particularly during those weeks in which we achieved the goal of zero facility-acquired pressure ulcers. We presented gift certificates and held parties for everything from the most improved unit to the unit that held the record for no new pressure ulcers.

Organizations undertaking a pilot such as the SKIN project at Ascension Health should expect a spike in the reported skin breakdown when the initiative is under way. As discussed earlier, such an increase in incidence is likely related to the staff's increased awareness, education, and reporting. The numbers will decrease with time. To further facilitate that downward trend, we considered other factors that may negatively affect pressure ulcer incidence, such as protocols that require patients to sit for several hours as part of a treatment regimen and areas in which patients may spend extended periods lying or sitting, such as radiology or dialysis. The SKIN team began to develop plans to provide pressure relief in these situations. Learning such as this was added to the changes spread to other facilities.

We found initial resistance from one physician to the medical staff's preapproved standing orders for dietitians. His concerns were successfully addressed one on one.

Another barrier observed was occasional patient and/or family reluctance to allow the SKIN bundle to be used. Further discussion revealed that the root cause of the hesitancy was a fear of pain for the patient during turning. With appropriate education and pain management, the SKIN bundle could be successfully implemented for these patients.

In addition to changing the treatment interventions, we learned that product reviews must be part of an initiative to eliminate facility-acquired pressure ulcers. Involving clinical staff, including WOCNs, helped us to analyze new or current skin care products and adjunctive equipment.

St. Vincent's continued to find patients with multiple comorbidities for whom skin breakdown occurred even when all aspects of the SKIN bundle were implemented. However, the goal of zero facility-acquired pressure ulcers is appropriate, attainable, and sustainable. In addition, a patient who arrives for treatment with a pressure ulcer should be discharged with no deterioration in the ulcer or, preferably, with documented improvement. A commitment to these goals has been a core component of the successful spread to other facilities within Ascension Health. At a recent meeting of the clinical leadership of Ascension Health, one CNO reported the devastation her staff felt when a facility-acquired pressure ulcer was discovered after nearly two years without one in that hospital.

Conclusion

Through a comprehensive program to reduce and eliminate facility-acquired pressure ulcers, St. Vincent's was free of Stage IV facility-acquired pressure ulcers from August 2004 to May 2007. The SKIN program has been shared, adopted, and successfully implemented in all 65 acute care hospitals of Ascension Health. The alpha site model and spread process used for the prevention of facility-acquired pressure ulcers is now being used for falls prevention, care of bariatric patients, and reduction of patient handling injuries.

References

1. Pryor D.B., et al.: The clinical transformation of Ascension Health: Eliminating preventable injuries and deaths. *Jt Comm J Qual Patient Saf* 32:299–308, Jun. 2006.
2. Wound Ostomy and Continence Nurses (WOCN) Society: *Clinical Practice Guideline Series: Guidelines for Prevention and Management of Pressure Ulcers.* Glenview, IL: WOCN Society, 2003.
3. Ratliff C.R., Rodeheaver G.T.: Pressure ulcer assessment and management. *Lippincott's Primary Care Practice* 3:242–258, Mar.–Apr. 1999.
4. Cuddigan J., Ayello E.A., Sussman C. (eds.).: *Pressure Ulcers in America: Prevalence, Incidence, and Implications for the Future.* Reston, VA: National Pressure Ulcer Advisory Panel, 2001.
5. Eckman K.: The prevalence of dermal ulcers among persons in the U.S. who have died. *Decubitus* 2:36–40, May 1989.
6. Hill-Rom: *Hill-Rom International Pressure Ulcer Prevalence Study.* Batesville, IN: Hill-Rom, 2007.
7. Allman R: The impact of pressure ulcers on healthcare costs and mortality. *Adv Wound Care* 11(3 Suppl.):2, May–Jun. 1998.
8. Beckrich K., Aronovitch S.: Hospital-acquired pressure ulcers: A comparison of costs in medical vs. surgical patients. *Nurs Econ* 17:263–271, Sep.–Oct. 1999.

9. Prevention Plus: *The Braden Scale for Predicting Pressure Sore Risk.* http://www.bradenscale.com/bradenscale.htm (accessed Jun. 26, 2006).

10. Hill-Rom: *Hill-Rom International Pressure Ulcer Prevalence Study.* Batesville, IN: Hill-Rom, 2004.

Chapter 3
Preventing Central Line–Associated Bloodstream Infections at Beth Israel Medical Center

Brian Koll, M.D.
Ina Jabara, R.N.
Kathy Peterson, R.N.
David Crimmins, R.N., C.I.C.
Alexis Raimondi, R.N., C.I.C.
Samuel Acquah, M.D.
Hosam Sayed, M.D.

Background and Overview

Beth Israel Medical Center is a two-hospital, not-for-profit, teaching 918-bed tertiary care center located in New York City. One hospital is located in Manhattan; the other is located in Brooklyn. Its two hospitals have seven intensive care units (ICUs) and two stepdown units. There are 94 ICU beds with 3,000 discharges and 824 non-ICU beds with 43,000 discharges annually; 2,500 central lines are placed yearly. Table 3-1 (page 42) compares Beth Israel Medical Center with other medical centers in the United States regarding central line use and central line–associated bloodstream infections (CLABs) in its adult ICUs—before the spread of the central line bundle.

Approximately 2 million health care–associated infections occur in hospitals in the United States annually, resulting in 90,000 deaths.[1] Infections with central venous catheters are a substantial problem. CLABs are the third-most-common health care–associated infection after ventilator-associated pneumonias and Foley catheter–associated urinary tract infections reported by medical-surgical ICUs participating in the Centers for Disease Control and Prevention's (CDC's) National Nosocomial Infection Surveillance System.[2] Each year, nearly 250,000 cases of CLABs occur in hospitals in the United States.[3]

Approximately 53% of adult patients in the ICU have a central venous catheter on any given day.[4] In the ICU, central venous catheters may be needed for extended periods of time, patients can be colonized with hospital-acquired organisms, and the catheter can be manipulated multiple times per day for the administration of medications, intravenous fluids, and blood products. Catheters can also be accessed numerous times per day for hemodynamic measurements and to obtain blood specimens for laboratory analysis, augmenting the potential for contamination and subsequent CLAB.[3] Because of these factors, the

Table 3-1.
CENTRAL LINE USE AND CENTRAL LINE–ASSOCIATED BLOODSTREAM INFECTIONS (CLABs) BEFORE USE OF THE CENTRAL LINE BUNDLE*

	BIMC	U.S.
Patients in ICU with central line	40%	48%
CLABs rate per 1,000 line days	4.5	5.3
CLABs rate per 100 patients	2%	4%
Increased LOS	5 days	14 days

*Increase in length of stay (LOS) is based on all patients with CLAB. BIMC, Beth Israel Medical Center; ICU, intensive care unit; LOS, length of stay. Sources for U.S. data: References 3 and 6–11. Used with permission.

risk of CLABs is higher in the ICU setting than in non-ICU settings.

Each year in the United States, approximately 80,000 patients in ICUs develop CLABs.[5] The overall attributable mortality of CLABs varies. Estimates range between 0% and 35%, depending on the patient population, definitions, pathogens, and study methodology.[3,6–10] Assuming an average CLAB rate of 5.3 per 1,000 catheter days in ICUs and an attributable mortality of 18%, as many as 28,000 ICU patients die of CLABs annually in the United States.[11]

CLABs often prolong hospitalization by 10 to 40 days.[6-7] The attributable cost per CLAB is between $35,000 and $56,000.[9,12] The annual cost of caring for patients with CLABs ranges from $296 million to $2.3 billion.[5]

Because of the impact of CLABs on morbidity and mortality, increased length of hospital stay, and attributable costs, it is in the interest of everyone to decrease the rate of CLABs and improve the quality of ICU care. CLABs are preventable. Updated recommendations for the prevention of CLABs were published by the hospital's infection control practices advisory committee (HICPAC) in 2002.[3] Evidence-based practices to decrease CLABs, known as the Institute for Healthcare Improvement–developed central line bundle,[13] are incorporated into these recommendations. Implementation of the bundle results in better outcomes than separate implementation of the bundle components. The key components of the central line bundle are shown in Table 3-2 (page 43).

Despite the evidence for using these interventions to reduce the incidence of CLABs and the resulting morbidity, mortality, and costs, a gap exists between best evidence and best practices.[11] Multifaceted interventions that help ensure compliance with the evidenced-based practices of the central line bundle have proven effective in nearly eliminating CLABs in a hospital and regional setting.[11,14]

In December 2004, Beth Israel Medical Center set the goal of preventing CLABs and CLAB-related deaths by spreading the implementation of the central line bundle for all

Table 3-2.
THE CENTRAL LINE BUNDLE

- Hand hygiene
- Maximal barrier precautions
- Chlorhexidine skin antisepsis
- Optimal catheter site selection, with subclavian vein as the preferred site for non-tunneled catheters
- Daily review of line necessity, with prompt removal of unnecessary lines

Used with permission.

patients requiring a central line. The goal was chosen on the basis of Beth Israel's annual review and risk analysis of infectious disease levels at the medical center. The initiative built on the epidemiological model promulgated by The Joint Commission's Standard IC 2.10[15]:

- The review identified CLAB as the infection risk.

- The goal was to have zero CLABs.

- The strategy was implementation of the central line bundle.

- Reevaluation of the program was to occur through feedback of infection data to staff using standard definitions described later in the text.

Aim of the Spread Initiative

The aim of the spread initiative was to prevent CLABs and deaths in all patients requiring central lines by implementing a set of evidence-based interventions known as the central line bundle. Our goal was to create a systemic model for change that could be used anywhere in the hospital and that would use existing staffing and financial resources to create a process that generates sustainable fixes instead of tolerating the status quo of workarounds that were constantly repeated. Frontline staff would be empowered to get the job done and would be held accountable for reliable performance of basic practices to prevent these infections by working as interdisciplinary teams and owning the process. The knowledge gained from this process would be shared with all.

The goal of eliminating CLABs was put forth by the infection control committee to the hospital leadership because of this infection's impact on morbidity and mortality, length of stay, and hospital finances and because there was evidence that multifaceted interventions to help ensure compliance with the evidence-based practices of the central line bundle have proven effective in nearly eliminating CLABs in the hospital setting.

Because evidence existed that reaching this goal could be done rather quickly if the project started small, senior leaders decided to begin the spread initiative in two units in the Manhattan hospital and one unit in the Brooklyn hospital. The aim was to achieve 100% compliance with practices to prevent CLABs within 60 days and elimination of this infection within 90 days. Within one year, we would spread the initiative throughout the medical center.

The spread initiative was a strategic priority for the hospital and fit in well with its leadership's goals for the medical center, which included delivery of quality care and services and increasing growth and improving finances through reduction of length of stay and improvment of efficiency.

Methods

Leadership Involvement

Medical center leadership was very important in effecting change. In December 2004, the chief executive officer, chief medical officer, and chief of infection control [B.K.] met with the medical directors and nursing leadership of each adult ICU to discuss the CLAB initiative and ensure that there were unit-based physician and nursing champions to support the initiative's goals of eliminating CLABs within 90 days. To get buy-in, education and review of the literature with these champions and their staff was important. The hospital epidemiologist [B.K.] then conducted a biweekly series of learning sessions, which were part didactic, part discussion, with clinicians and nonclinicians for these ICUs during the next four months. The learning sessions, which involved discussion of successful initiatives outside New York, were designed to persuade the participants to believe that *hospital factors specific to the medical center had a greater influence on infection risk than a patient's severity of illness.* In the learning sessions, each unit was asked to define what the problems were in relation to CLABs and how best to solve these problems. The hospital epidemiologist served as the promoter of the spread initiative, working with the physician and nursing champions and providing encouragement and reinforcement.

Developing Successful Sites: Unit-Based Teams

In January 2005, the medical ICU and the surgical ICU at the Manhattan hospital and the medical-surgical ICU at the Brooklyn hospital were chosen as the initial units to quickly implement the central line bundle. The medical and surgical ICUs at the Manhattan hospital are staffed by residents in training, fellows, and attendings. The medical-surgical ICU at the Brooklyn hospital is staffed by attending intensivists. The CLAB infection rate of the ICU at the Brooklyn hospital was higher than the CDC's National Healthcare Safety Network (NHSN) benchmarks; the medical ICU and surgical ICU at the Manhattan hospital had infection rates at the NHSN benchmark. Each unit had a physician and nursing champion and staff eager to improve the care of their patients. Each unit thought that its patients were "different and sicker than others" so that if infection rates could be reduced in these "sickest" patients, then buy-in elsewhere in the medical center would be made easier when it was decided to spread the initiative to another unit. Each unit posed related but different challenges that would need to be addressed systemically to allow spread elsewhere in the medical center. Because the infection rate at the Brooklyn ICU was the highest of the three, we started there before spreading to the other two ICUs. It was felt that the patients in this ICU were the sickest of the three and, as noted before, that if we could institute change here, resistance elsewhere would lessen considerably.

Unit-based multidisciplinary teams were created, each composed of ICU physicians, nursing staff, infection control pro-

Table 3-3. MULTIDISCIPLINARY CENTRAL LINE–ASSOCIATED BLOODSTREAM INFECTION (CLAB) PRINCIPLES

- It is not good enough that our infection rates are below national benchmarks.
- CLABs are preventable; they are not an inevitable consequence of sophisticated, complex care that we provide to our severely ill patients.
- CLABs can be eliminated through determination as opposed to additional resources.

Used with permission.

fessionals, interns, and residents, as well as representatives from other important departments, such as emergency medicine, nursing education, and materials management. Inclusion of other departments, such as emergency medicine, and physicians in training was important to help promote spread of the central line bundle and ensure sustainability.

To effect change in a rapid manner, each team developed three basic principles, as shown in Table 3-3 (above). The multidisciplinary teams met weekly to quickly implement the central line bundle using the plan-do-study-act (PDSA) methodology[16] (Figure 3-1, page 45) and achieve the goal of zero CLABs. This was accomplished through the following practices and activities:

1. Standardization of practices to ensure use of maximal barrier protection, preparation of skin with chlorhexidine, and preference for the subclavian site unless medically contraindicated.

2. Development of a central line insertion kit that contained barrier precaution, insertion, and maintenance

Figure 3-1.
PLAN-DO-STUDY-ACT METHODOLOGY

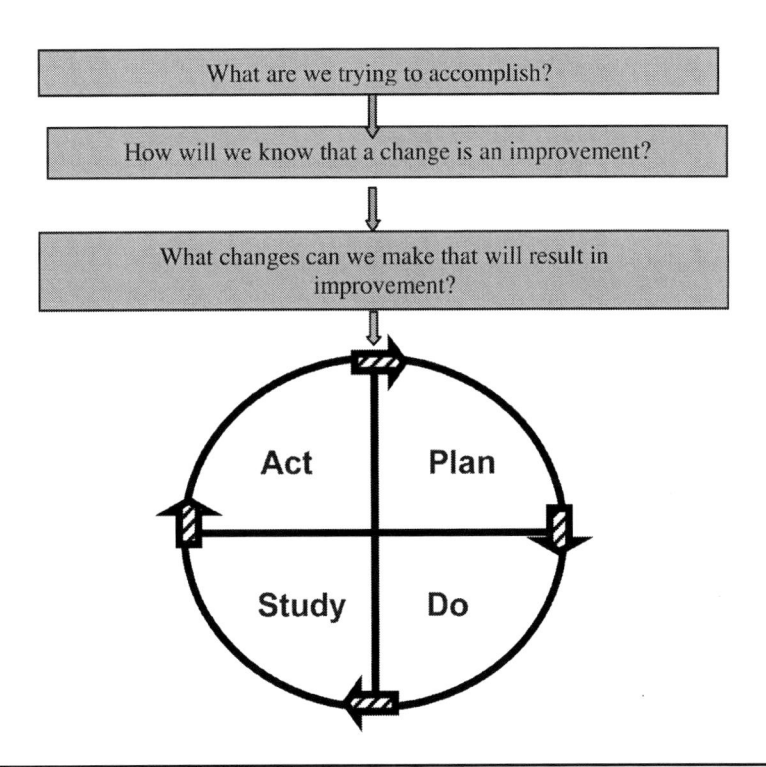

```
What are we trying to accomplish?
            ↓
How will we know that a change is an improvement?
            ↓
What changes can we make that will result in
                improvement?
            ↓
         [Act | Plan]
         [Study | Do]
```

The plan-do-study-act methodology, as part of the Model for Improvement, is shown. Source: Langley G.J., et al.: The Improvement Guide: A Practical Approach to Enhancing Organizational Performance. *San Francisco: Jossey-Bass, 1996. Used with permission.*

components. The involvement of materials management was extremely important in developing and implementing these kits. The kits (Figure 3-2, page 46) ensured that all needed supplies for compliance with the central line bundle were readily available and easily attainable.

3. Physician and nurse reeducation and recertification on central line insertion technique and maintenance practices.

4. Nursing empowerment to monitor practices. Nursing staff already played a key role in ensuring hand-hygiene compliance. As they did for hand hygiene, nurses were permitted to ask and stop physicians who did not follow the central line bundle.

5. Daily bedside interdisciplinary rounds to include review of central line necessity and ensure removal of unnecessary lines.

6. Root cause analyses (RCAs) performed in real time for every CLAB.

An RCA was conducted within 24 hours of each CLAB. The 4 to 12 persons who were involved in the care of the patient—ICU, non-ICU, and emergency department staff—participated. The RCAs, which each lasted about 30 to 45 minutes, were collaborative and nonpunitive. Each RCA was expected to result in a solution for each CLAB that would generate a sustainable fix and avoid workarounds that are consistently repeated. One workaround that was

Figure 3-2.
CENTRAL LINE KIT

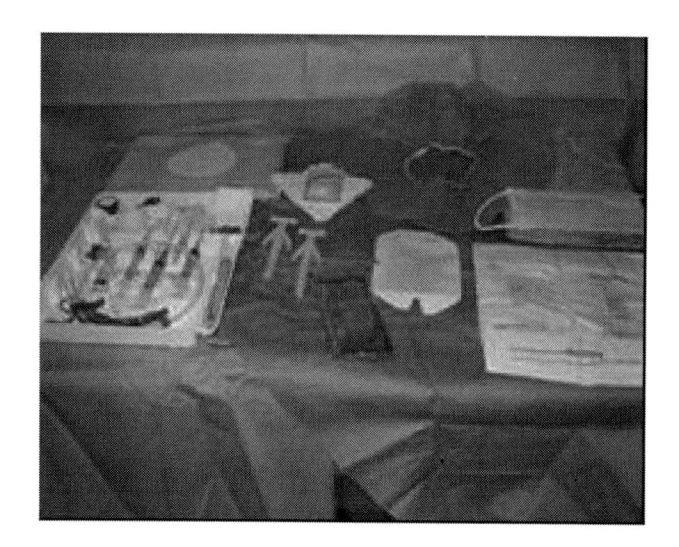

Barrier and Maintenance Components

- Cap
- Mask
- Gown
- Sterile gloves
- Extra-large fenestrated drape
- Alcohol swabs
- Preoperative swab prep (2% chlorhexidine gluconate, 70% isopropyl alcohol)
- Tincture of benzoine
- Large transparent dressing
- Biopatch
- Tape/securement device

Insertion Components

- Indwelling catheter
- Spring-wire guide
- Catheter
- Injection needles (safety engineered)
- Introducer needle (safety engineered)
- Syringes
- Tissue dilator
- Clamp
- Fastener
- Sterilization wrap
- Scalpel (safety engineered)
- Gauze pads
- Suture materials
- Prefilled saline flush
- Lidocaine

The central line kit is shown in the photo; barrier and maintenance components and insertion components are listed. Used with permission.

consistently mentioned was the lack of easy access to supplies necessary to insert a central line. Staff had to go from room to room, cabinet to cabinet, to get everything together. This took a fair amount of time, and there was room for error if something could not be found. A central line cart was created to help solve this problem. Unfortunately, there were stocking issues, such as incorrect sizes of gloves and incorrect drapes. To solve this problem, a central line kit was ultimately created that contained all necessary supplies and was easily accessible. The end users (those placing the lines) worked with materials management to create the kits. The end users needed to be involved because they would be using the components of the kit, and if they did not like what was in the kit, then the functionality and usefulness of the kit would have been negated. The knowledge gained from each RCA was shared with everyone.

In addition to helping identify the need for and ultimately the creation of the central line kit, the RCAs were an important component in empowering nurses to enforce the central line bundle. For example, at the beginning of the initiative, a physician was not following the bundle, but nursing staff were nervous about confronting her. She would not abide by the nurse's entreaties, and ultimately, the nurse and her supervisor called the physician's director, who supported their efforts and stopped the procedure. Two days later, when the patient became fungemic, the nursing staff felt vindicated but also were upset that they had not been more assertive. They felt that if they had been, the infection might have been prevented. The RCA for this infection was conducted by the physician in question, who recognized that she should have respected the nurses, better understood the importance of the central line bundle for prevention of infection, and also have devised a corrective action plan. The support that was given to the nurses and the fact that physicians were doing their own RCAs and coming up with corrective actions were very important in changing culture and letting everyone see how important this campaign was. A change in culture was also evident in health care workers' apparent comfort in stopping one another if hand hygiene was not performed, the introduction of bedside multidisciplinary rounding teams, and improved communication between caregivers. The involvement of materials management was also an important reminder to all that nonclinicians play major roles in reducing infections and improving patient safety and delivery of care.

Data Collection
The CDC's NHSN definition of CLAB was used. Each ICU reported on the number of patients with a central line and the number of central line days for each patient. Infection control professionals collected data on the number of CLABs. Compliance with the central line bundle was documented using a standardized vascular procedure note, as shown in Figure 3-3 (page 48). CLAB infection data and compliance with the central line bundle were reported to the individual units on a monthly basis.

Results in Initial Sites

Implementation of the central line bundle and reduction of CLABs was achieved in the initial three units within 90 days. As shown in Figure 3-4 (page 49), the surgical ICU at the Manhattan hospital achieved a rate of 0 CLABs per 1,000 line days after implementation of the central line bundle.

Spread of Central Line Bundle to Other Units

Shortly after implementation of the central line bundle and reduction of CLABs in the initial three units, spread to other areas of the hospital occurred in rapid succession, using the PDSA methodology. In June 2005, a communication plan that included a time frame to spread to other areas of the hospital was carried out. Every month, data from the initial three units were shared with the staff of these units and with the board of trustees, hospital administration, nursing leadership, physician leadership, the residency training program, nonclinical staff, and other patient care units through a variety of methods, including a hospitalwide newsletter, electronic e-mail, and posters and in-services at departmental meetings and grand rounds. In-services were provided by the chief of infection control, physician and nursing champions, and, ultimately, critical care unit staff. The plan for spread of the initiative is shown in Table 3-4 (page 49). The timing for spread to other areas during the year was based on where buy-in had already occurred (as reflected in results for the initial three units) or where resistance to spread was minimal. Reduction of CLABs in the non-ICU areas of the Brooklyn hospital are shown in Figure 3-5 (page 50). As is evident from the figure, the rate of reduction in CLABs was very similar for

Figure 3-3.
CENTRAL LINE–ASSOCIATED BLOODSTREAM INFECTION (CLAB) MONITORING TOOL

BETH ISRAEL MEDICAL CENTER
VASCULAR ACCESS PROCEDURE NOTE

Date: _____
Time Out at _____ AM/PM
Verified Correct (all must be verified):   ✓ Patient   ✓ Procedure   ✓ Site/Side
✓ Position   ✓ Supplies   ✓ Equipment

_____ RN/MD   _____ RN/MD

Central vein: ✓ R   ✓ L
Pulmonary artery: ✓ R   ✓ L
Transvenous pacemaker: ✓ R   ✓ L
✓ subclavian ✓ internal jugular   ✓ femoral (if femoral, reason for choice) _____

Arterial: ✓ R   ✓ L   ✓ radial   ✓ femoral   ✓ other_____

Indication(s): _____

Consent in chart ✓   Operator(s): _____

Central Line Check List:	
1- ✓ All equipments at bedside	8 - ✓ Time-out
2- ✓ Wash hands	9 - ✓ Mask
3- ✓ Chlor- prep	10 - ✓ Procedure with sterile technique
4- ✓ Gown	11 - ✓ Bio-Patch
5- ✓ Gloves	12 - ✓ Dressing with date
6- ✓ Cap	13 - ✓ Dispose sharps
7- ✓ Drape	14 - ✓ Wash hands

Anesthesia: _____

Technique: _____

Comments: _____

Complications: _____

_____
Signature/Title
Time: _____

Compliance with the central line bundle was documented as performed using a standardized vascular procedure note. Used with permission.

Figure 3-4.
RATE OF CENTRAL LINE–ASSOCIATED BLOODSTREAM INFECTIONS (CLABs) PER 1,000 LINE DAYS AT BETH ISRAEL MEDICAL-SURGICAL ICU: MANHATTAN HOSPITAL, 2004–2006

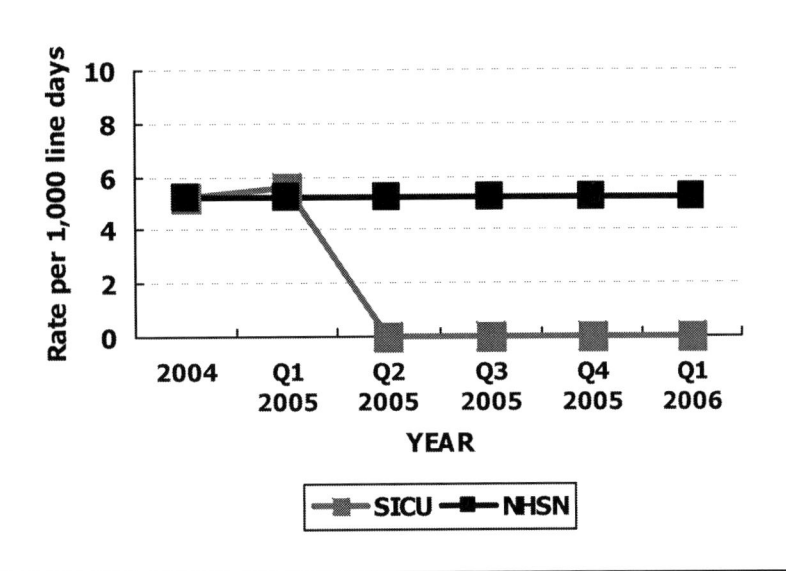

The surgical intensive care unit (ICU) at the Manhattan hospital achieved a rate of zero CLABs per 1,000 line days after implementation of the central line bundle. The mean rate of 4.9 CLABs for the three ICUs, as provided by the National Healthcare Safety Network (NHSN), is shown. Used with permission.

Table 3-4.
BETH ISRAEL MEDICAL CENTER TIME LINE FOR CLABs SPREAD*

- January 2005
  — Manhattan hospital: medical ICU, surgical ICU
  — Brooklyn hospital: medical-surgical ICU

- August 2005
  — Manhattan hospital: cardiac ICU and cardiac surgery ICU

- December 2005
  — Emergency departments

- January 2006
  — Brooklyn hospital: General medical-surgical and stepdown units

- April 2006
  — Brooklyn hospital: operating room
  — Manhattan hospital: general medical-surgical and stepdown units

- August 2006
  — Manhattan hospital pediatric ICU

*ICU, intensive care unit. Used with permission.

> **Figure 3-5.**
> **RATE OF NON-INTENSIVE CARE UNIT (ICU) CENTRAL LINE–ASSOCIATED BLOODSTREAM INFECTIONS (CLABS) PER 1,000 LINE DAYS AT BETH ISRAEL MEDICAL CENTER: BROOKLYN HOSPITAL, 2006.**
>
> *The rate of reduction in CLABs at the Brooklyn hospital was very similar to that of the initial ICUs. Used with permission.*

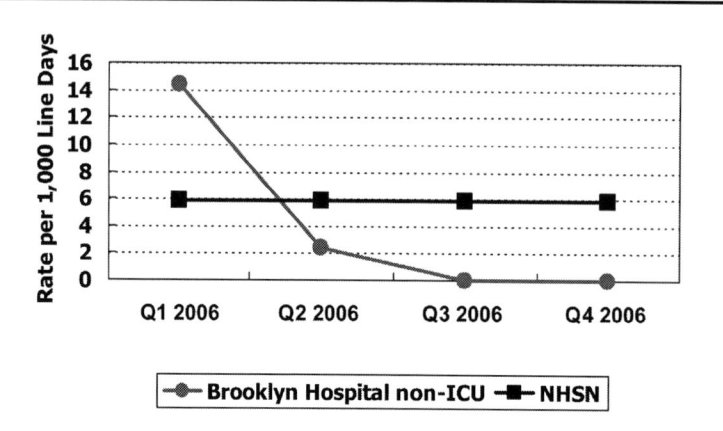

the initial ICUs and the other areas of the medical center to which the initiative was spread.

One area where buy-in was difficult was the neonatal ICU. The neonatologists were reluctant to adopt and modify for neonates practices that were originally developed for adults. Consequently, their unit was one of the last units included in the spread. Our "window of opportunity" came when they had a spate of infections. Although the rates were below NHSN benchmarks, the neonatologists believed in the concept of "zero infections" and were finally ready to join the initiative and allow spread.

System Results
For each unit where the spread occurred, 100% compliance with the central line bundle took about 60 days. Once 100% compliance was achieved, it was sustained for more than one year. Compliance data for one ICU is shown in Figure 3-6 (page 51). Across the Beth Israel Medical Center, the CLAB rate per 1,000 central line days decreased from 4.5 to 1.2 and is below the NHSN rate of 4.9. The CLAB rate per 100 patients with a central line decreased from 2% to 0.6% and is below that reported in the literature of 4% (Figure 3-7, page 51). The three units achieved a median of 307 days without a CLAB. Reduction in central line days, lives saved, and costs avoided through prevention of CLABs is shown in Table 3-5 (page 52). The longest duration of days without a CLAB for the ICUs and stepdown units following implementation of the central line bundle is shown in Table 3-6 (page 52).

Lessons Learned and Next Steps

Consistent use and monitoring of evidence-based patient care practices, or "bundles," with reporting back of data to end users resulted in the rapid and sustained elimination or decreased incidence of CLABs at Beth Israel Medical Center. The PDSA methodology[15] was applicable across two hospitals in a variety of units. Support of hospital leadership and identification of physician and nursing champions was the key to the rapid and sustained success.

Figure 3-6.
COMPLIANCE WITH CENTRAL LINE BUNDLE, AUGUST 2005–DECEMBER 2006

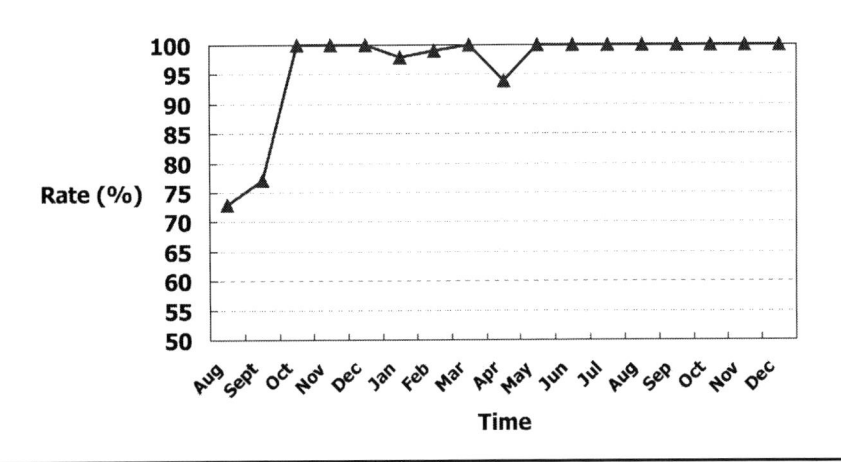

One intensive care unit's rate of compliance in terms of compliance by line insertion with the central line bundle is shown. Used with permission.

Figure 3-7.
CENTRAL LINE–ASSOCIATED BLOODSTREAM INFECTION (CLAB) RATE, 2004–2006.

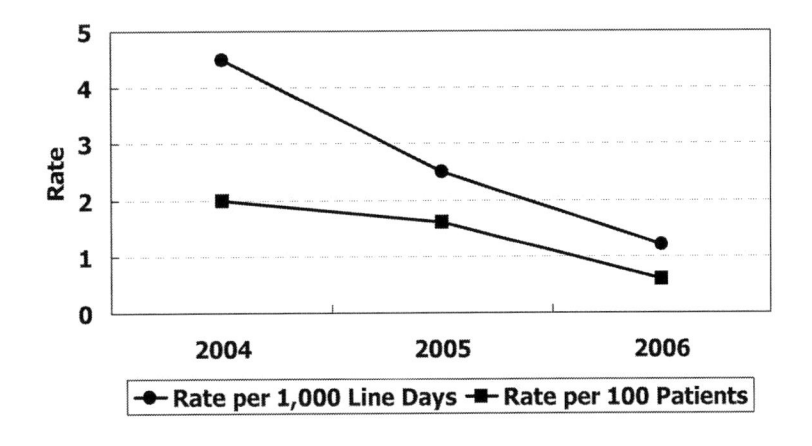

Across the Beth Israel Medical Center, the CLAB rate per 1,000 central line days decreased from 4.5% to 1.2%, and the CLAB rate per 100 patients with a central line decreased from 2% to 0.6%. Used with permission.

Table 3-5.
BENEFITS OF THE CENTRAL–LINE ASSOCIATED BLOODSTREAM INFECTION (CLAB) INITIATIVE, 2004–2006

- 83% reduction in CLABs
- 31% decrease in central line days
- 10 lives saved
- Reduction of $1,330,000 in costs involved in caring for patients with CLABs
- Costs to implement:
  — Additional $15 per line inserted
  — Creation of a central line insertion kit: an additional $37,500

Used with permission.

Table 3-6.
LONGEST DURATION OF DAYS WITHOUT A CENTRAL LINE–ASSOCIATED BLOODSTREAM INFECTION (CLAB) FOLLOWING CENTRAL LINE BUNDLE IMPLEMENTATION AS OF DECEMBER 31, 2006*

Unit	Maximum Days Without CLAB
Cardiac ICU	432
Surgical ICU	431
Emergency Room	396
Medical-Surgical ICU	387
Pediatric ICU	274
Cardiac Surgery ICU	274
Neonatal ICU	255
Surgical Stepdown	245
Non-ICU	240
Medical ICU	213
Respiratory Stepdown	167

ICU, intensive care unit. Used with permission.

Limited additional resources were necessary for the success of this initiative. Culture change regarding the goal of zero CLABs was evident for this device-related infection and can indeed be achieved for all other hospital-acquired infections and patient safety issues. Similar initiatives are already under way at Beth Israel for eliminating infections due to methicillin-resistant *Staphylococcus aureus* and *Clostridium difficile*—with the same spread techniques as used for CLABs. As before, Beth Israel is starting in the medical ICU of the Manhattan hospital and the medical-surgical ICU of the Brooklyn hospital. It is also including orthopedic and cardiac surgeons initially because *S. aureus* infections are seen in these services with devastating consequences. Whereas materials management played an important role in the creation of the central line insertion kit, housekeeping and transporters are playing key roles in the elimination of infections due to methicillin-resistant *S. aureus* and *C. difficile;* they are creating special environmental protocols for cleaning of equipment and rooms. As before, data are regularly shared with all.

References

1. Weinstein R.A.: Nosocomial infection update. *Emerg Infect Dis* 4:416–420, Jul.–Sep. 1998.
2. Richards M.J., et al.: Nosocomial infections in combined medical-surgery intensive care units in the United States. *Infect Control Hosp Epidemiol* 21:510–515, May 1999.
3. Miller D.L., O'Grady N.P.: Guidelines for the prevention of intravascular catheter related infections. *Am J Infect Control* 30:476–489, Dec. 2002.
4. National Nosocomial Infections Surveillance (NNIS) system report, data summary from January 1992–April 2000, issued June 2000. *Am J Infect Control* 28:429–448, Dec. 2000.
5. Mermel L.A.: Prevention of intravascular catheter-related infections. *Ann Intern Med* 7:391–402, Mar. 2000.
6. Pittet D., et al.: Nosocomial bloodstream infection in critically ill patients: Excess length of stay, extra costs, and attributable mortality. *JAMA* 271:1598–1601, May 25, 1994.
7. Digiovine B., et al.: The attributable mortality and costs of primary nosocomial bloodstream infections in the intensive care unit. *Am J Respir Crit Care Med* 160:976–981, Sep. 1999.
8. Soulfir L., et al.: Attributable morbidity and mortality of catheter-related septicemia in critically ill patients: A matched, risk-adjusted, cohort study. *Infect Control Hosp Epidemiol* 20:396–401, Jun. 1999.
9. Rello J., et al.: Evaluation of outcome of intravenous catheter-related infections in critically ill patients. *Am J Respir Crit Care Med* 162:1027–1030, Sep. 2000.
10. Rupp M.E., et al.: Effect of a second-generation venous catheter impregnated with chlorhexidine and silver sulfadiazine on central catheter-related infections. *Ann Intern Med* 143:570–580, Oct. 2005.
11. Berenholtz S.M., et al.: Eliminating catheter-related bloodstream infections in the intensive care unit. *Crit Care Med* 32:2014–2020, Oct. 2004.
12. Dimick J.B., et al.: Increased resource use associated with catheter-related bloodstream infection in the surgical intensive care unit. *Arch Surg* 136:229–234, Feb. 2001.
13. Institute for Healthcare Improvement: *Getting Started Kit: Prevent Central Line Infections. How-to Guide.* http://www.ihi.org/IHI/Programs/Campaign/Campaign.htm?TabId=2#PreventCentralLine-AssociatedBloodstreamInfection (accessed Sep. 10, 2007).
14. Centers for Disease Control and Prevention: Reduction in central line–associated bloodstream infections among patients in intensive care units—Pennsylvania. *MMWR Morb Mortal Wkly Rep* 54:1013–1016, Oct. 14, 2005.
15. The Joint Commission: *2007 Comprehensive Accreditation Manual for Hospital: The Official Handbook.* Oakbrook Terrace, IL: Joint Commission Resources, 2006.
16. Langley G.J., et al.: *The Improvement Guide.* San Francisco: Jossey-Bass, 1996.

Chapter 4:
Spreading the Nurse Knowledge Exchange Handoff Practices at Kaiser Permanente

Lisa Schilling, R.N., M.P.H.
Chris McCarthy, M.B.A., M.P.H.

Background and Overview

Kaiser Permanente (KP) is the largest nonprofit health plan in the United States, encompassing the not-for-profit Kaiser Foundation Health Plan Inc., Kaiser Foundation Hospitals and their subsidiaries, and the for-profit Permanente Medical Groups, as well as an affiliation with the Seattle-based Group Health Cooperative. There are 135,000 employees and 13,000 Permanente physicians providing services in eight regions across the United States.

KP has leadership at the board level for the health plan, with nonvoting representatives from the medical group. Hospitals operate within regions and local delivery systems, each system with its own leadership, and report to the national board. This reporting structure, along with the organizational value of local autonomy for innovation, presents a challenge to any initiative in which a single practice is to be spread throughout the delivery system.

In this chapter, we [the KP program office team] describe the process used to develop and spread a handoff practice for nurses' shift change at Kaiser Permanente. This effort evolved as follows:

- January 2004: Initiation of innovation work with an innovation design consulting firm

- June 2004–December 2004: One hospital from each of the four regions that has KP-owned inpatient facilities designs and pilots practices that result in the Nurse Knowledge Exchange (NKE) handoff practice.

- January 2005–August 2005: Support sustainability of initial pilot sites, hold leadership discussion for spread, refine and finalize change package

- August 2005: Decision to spread the practice

- December 2005: Final launch of spread through formation of a KP-wide collaborative

- December 2006: Completion across 20 hospitals

In 2005, KP, in collaboration with the Institute for Healthcare Improvement (IHI), decided to use a set of nurse shift-change handoff practices, known as NKE, to test a new method for spreading an improvement in a uniform manner within a specific time period—nine months from launching the first group of units. Given the value given of autonomy for innovating change, we structured this spread effort in the context of building will among hospitals and staff, creating a shared vision by involving nursing executives at the regional and hospital levels, and developing a communication plan with hospital leadership teams. We began our spread effort at the end of the innovation pilot phase of the practice. In August 2005 we convened a group of nursing and quality leaders from across Kaiser Permanente and met with spread experts from IHI to determine the scope and scale of the spread effort. Once we identified the hospitals that would engage in spreading NKE as a practice, we were able to engage them in the design, sponsorship, and communication strategy for implementation.

The Problem of Nurse Shift Change

Before NKE was developed, at shift change in medical centers across the KP system, each nurse had his or her own way of gathering and maintaining incredibly complex amounts of patient information during the shift. At shift change, the nurse shared this information verbally, using his or her own checklist and a tape-recorded shift report that all oncoming nurses listened to for a system-by-system (for example, cardiovascular, respiratory) review of each patient. Each unit in each hospital had a preferred way of supporting nurses' shift-change communications, such as communicating assignments and patient information.

In an ideal situation, handoff at shift change would provide a seamless transition in a patient's care because the nurse typically would have a clear care plan and good organizational skills and, on the basis of experience, know what information is important to transfer. However, gathering and maintaining this information took up a significant part of the nurse's shift work, and there was a good chance that this information would be lost, forgotten, or "miscommunicated." Yet, interviews and observation suggested that nurses often gathered the information they "really needed" *after* report by reviewing patients' charts and talking with other care providers and the patients, which suggests that the report was not effective.

By early 2004, a number of other factors had come together to make nurse shift change a process ripe for innovation, including the arrival at KP of the electronic health record (EHR)—KP HealthConnect—and the 2006 Joint Commission National Patient Goals. NKE, described in the next section, helped prepare the unit for the impending implementation of the EHR by increasing proficiency in personal computer use and optimizing work flows. NKE also addressed The Joint Commission National Patient Safety Goals regarding handoff practices* and patient and family involvement.[†,1]

NKE: A Change-of-Shift Innovation

Developing NKE

In January 2004, KP partnered with a design consulting firm specializing in innovation and "transformation" to ask staff and leaders from the four hospital regions where KP owned hospitals, "Within the hospital, where are the opportunities for innovation?" These four regions identified nurses' shift change as a process that could be innovated in a way that is patient centered and staff friendly and helps pave the way for an EHR implementation.

In the assessment phase, we performed site visits to the pilot units in each facility and engaged frontline staff in the process, asking them to determine which work flows or processes were most challenging to them. The top two answers were nurse communication at shift change and bed management, which was the most compelling reason for the innovation initiative to focus on a new system for nurse handoffs at shift change.

KP recognized that the process of nurse communication at shift change was similar to processes in other high-reliability industries, such as nuclear power, aviation, and nuclear submarine systems. Requiring face-to-face handoffs with a structured report tool and engaging all members in the report during handoffs is a common practice in such industries.[2] We had placed a strategic safety focus on reliable design, so we adopted several of these safety principles in designing the reliable handoff practice.

The innovation method used consists of five basic steps: observation, storytelling, brainstorming, prototyping, and

---

*2E: "Implement a standardized approach to 'hand off' communications, including an opportunity to ask and respond to questions."

†13: "Encourage the active involvement of patients and their families in the patient's care as a patient safety strategy" and 13A: "Define and communicate the means for patients to report concerns about safety and encourage them to do so."

field testing. "Ghost town" and "The need to prepare" were two of the signature stories that came out of the observation/storytelling with staff. Oncoming charge nurses typically felt the need to arrive 30 to 45 minutes before their official shift start time to prepare for the oncoming staff. During this time, a charge nurse would get a "feel for the floor," confirm staffing plans, organize the work tasks for oncoming certified nursing assistants, and finally oversee shift report. Yet at the same time, oncoming staff needed to start answering patient requests before they had the information they needed to provide appropriate care.

Patients and providers worried about the decrease in attention to patient care at shift change. One patient characterized the unit as a "ghost town," and many providers said it was "chaos," with all the administrative needs having to be taken care of while patient calls, orders, laboratory test results, and other demands continued to pour in.

In the brainstorming phase, more than 400 ideas were generated, which the prototyping phase narrowed to fewer than 10. Finally, the field-testing phase refined the ideas to what it now known as the four-step practice of NKE.

NKE in Detail

NKE is a system of practices that is composed of the following primary components:

- *Bedside rounds:* Oncoming and outgoing nurses conduct shift change at the bedside and use the communication technique known as "patient teach-back" with the patient and family, as appropriate. This technique addresses health literacy issues in a patient care population and is a core aspect of the NKE change package. Bedside rounds reduce the time from the nurse's arrival on a unit to when he or she physically see the patient. This is the foundation of the NKE system.

- *Patient goal board:* Oncoming nurses write shift goals that are easily understood by the patient on a visible whiteboard. For example, a nurse would write "walk the hallway three times today" instead of "ambulate 3X."

- *Previous shift prep:* The outgoing charge nurse prepares the nurse-patient assignments for the oncoming shift. The oncoming charge nurse confirms the assignments and prepares for unit hand off.

- *Structured report:* This tool, either electronic or paper based, assists the oncoming nurse in structured focused communication about the issues, plans, needs, and potential safety issues for each patient when preparing for shift change. The data template contains all the basic patient data that nurses need for safe and efficient handoff. An example of a paper data template used at one hospital is shown in Figure 4-1 (page 58). The computer template incorporated into the EHR system, as shown in Figure 4-2 (page 59), combines user-friendly electronic record-keeping with a seamless personal handoff of each patient from one caregiver to the next. It represents a more efficient way for nurses to share information about patients at the change of shift. KP HealthConnect is being implemented in all KP hospitals and outpatient clinics.

NKE enables a nurse shift change that has the following characteristics:

- *Member centered:* The process is warm and friendly for the patients and families.

- *Patient safe:* Handoffs are verbal, face-to-face, use standardized tools and language (such as Identification-Situation-Background-Assessment-Recommendation [iSBAR][3] [Figure 4-3, page 60]) and consider concepts of reliable design.

- *Team centered:* The process increases the strength of the team across shifts.

- *Efficient:* Nurses are "ready to go" on arrival (no waiting for assignments).

- *Focused:* Nurses prepare and receive only their patients (not the whole unit) and use a report tool to focus on critical information.

Figure 4-1.

Sample Paper Data Template for Shift Report

SHIFT REPORT

DATE:__________ CODE STATUS: __________ Anticipated D/C Date:__________

DX: __________

Surgery/Date: __________

Pt History: __________

Allergies:__________

Patient Sticker

NOT PART OF THE PERMANENT PATIENT RECORD

	DAYS	PMs	NOCs
ACTIVE PROBLEMS (PROBLEM/GOAL LIST)			
TELE RHYTHM			
PAIN LEVEL # PAIN MEASURES			
DIET ACCUδ/ASSISTANCE			
MOBILITY/ACTIVITY FOR SHIFT ASSISTIVE DEVICES:			
RISK FACTORS/SAFETY RESTRAINTS : WRIST/ POSEY/ MITTENS			
IV LINES DATE LINE/DRESSING TO BE CHANGED:			
WOUND CARE/PRESSURE ULCERS			
RESPIRATORY/O_2			
TUBES/DRAINS			
LAST BM			
PENDING LABS/PROCEDURES ★TRANSFUSIONS			
REFFERALS MADE			
SOCIAL/SPECIAL NEEDS/MISC. FAMILY NEEDS			
	Report by:	Report by:	Report by:

Sample paper data template used in one hospital is shown. Used with permission.

Through implementing NKE in all inpatient care units, KP planned to improve patient satisfaction and staff satisfaction and reduce incidents involving harm, such as injuries from patient falls, through improvements in communication among the care team and recognition of patient risk.

Research through observation in the innovation phase showed many variations—not just across hospitals but across units and even within units. For example, in one unit, most nurses used a tape recorder to record their shift change information; however, a few nurses were notoriously late for the recording, so they habitually gave verbal reports. The result was two different work flows "colliding" at shift change. Redesigning and maintaining work flows with respect to the EHR on the basis of this disjointed model would be extraordinarily complex and expensive.

NKE as High-Tech but "People Soft"

NKE simplifies and standardizes the shift change work flow, permitting an easier integration and implementation of the EHR while still focusing the shift change on the nurse–patient relationship. The data template used for the NKE was imported into the EHR so that the nurses were already familiar with the work flow and were already accustomed to gathering and reporting the same information.

Finally, in early 2004, the KP Model of Care, also known as the Caring Model, was reconceptualized as a "human-centered" design. That is, we redesigned tools, roles, spaces,

Figure 4-2.
COMPUTER TEMPLATE "NEURON" SHIFT REPORT TOOL

RN: Ametess Martin		
Room 201	Doe1, DANIEL (55, M)	MD: Eron / RN: Ametess Martin / Previous RN Estrella
	MRN: 12 Language: English	
Admit Date 3/31/2005	Dx: Peritonitis	**PROJECTED DISCHARGE**
	Hx: HTN, ESRD, CAPD	Date / Time
Day 0	Surgery:	Dest Home / Trans UNKNOWN
	Isolation: None	Contact / Phone
CODE FULL	Allergies	Barriers
	Assistance OOB w/assist	Drains: CAPD Q 6 hrs. 2.5% alternate 1.5% all 2.5 liters
	Fall Risk: Medium	
Acuity 3	Diet: Renal	Labs: 3/31 Am
	Vital Frequency q4	
	Weight: Daily Weigh on empty	
	02: Yes	
	I/O: Yes Limit:	
	PCA Med: None	Additional Comments: c/c abd painx2days, no N/V. CT Abd done@ER. NO SBO. Abd slt dist/soft. Tenkoff site no redness. No reports of nausea, has cramping(epigastric) Pain 6/10 Med. C MS 2mg. & bloating. Effluent is cloudy,lrg fibrin, specimen sent @ 1100
	IVF HL	
	BS: None	

The computer template in the electronic health record system is shown. The term neuron *was chosen to reflect the tool's intended use as an extension of the user's brain. Used with permission.*

and processes with respect to our patients and care team. NKE addressed this strategy by focusing shift change on the nurse–patient relationship.

Aim of the Spread Initiative

KP's aim was to implement NKE on medical-surgical units in 20 hospitals by using a defined spread methodology, with work to be completed within nine months of the kickoff date (December 2006).

KP tested the innovation in the four pilot sites across the inpatient regions. Each site, selected by the sole criterion of its designation as the alpha site for the EHR in its respective region, was invited into the innovation project, and each accepted the invitation. Selection of the pilot unit was left as the hospital's choice; however, the unit had to be recognized as average or outstanding in its culture and performance.

At the end of the pilot, nurses and patients expressed a high degree of satisfaction with the NKE. Nurses liked having the structured report templates at the start of their shift and the ability to directly ask questions of the outgoing nurses; patients appreciated being involved in the bedside rounds component of the shift change and meeting the oncoming nurse. One of the four pilot sites did not complete the pilot process because of staffing and other issues. Nurses got to

> **Figure 4-3.**
> ## iSBAR: Modification of the Situation-Background-Assessment-Recommendation (SBAR) Tool
>
> - **I** – Identify yourselves, the patient
> - **S** – What are the 2-3 major issues on the table?
> - **B** – What do we know, what is pending?
> - **A** – Where are we?
> - **R** – What needs to be fixed, what does success look like?
>
> *The iSBAR tool was developed at Kaiser Permanente by Doug Bonacum. The SBAR Toolkit can be found at http://www.ihi.org/IHI/Topics/PatientSafety/SafetyGeneral/Tools/SBARToolkit.htm (accessed Jul. 12, 2007). Used with permission.*

see their patients three times faster using NKE, as demonstrated in Figure 4-4 (page 61). We did not include these measures during spread because the data collection was too cumbersome; instead, we decided to use incidental overtime as a proxy for time during shift change.

In August 2005, when we were planning to spread this practice to as many hospitals as possible, we used the results from the pilot sites to establish four outcome measures and several process measures. The outcome measures were as follows:

1. *Falls with injury (days between falls at the unit level).* This measure was chosen based on the knowledge that risk scoring systems and preventive interventions reduce risk for falls in the inpatient population. NKE as a practice would be used to clearly communicate fall risk and prevention activities.

2. *Patient satisfaction.* Three items from a patient survey, the Hospital Consumer Assessment of Healthcare Providers and Systems (H-CAHPS),[4] are called the nursing communication composite. These items are as follows: "nurses treated me with courtesy and respect," "nurses explained things in a way that I can understand," and "nurses listened carefully to me."

3. *Two staff satisfaction items from internal staff surveys.* These items, which address whether management values staff and team safety, are as follows: "everyone works together to ensure safety" and "when employees have good ideas about improving quality, management usually makes use of them."

4. *A financial measure for reduction in incidental overtime.* Pilot site results (Figure 4-4) indicated a significant reduction in the time it takes to see the first patient at change of shift.

Plan to Spread NKE

We considered the NKE pilot program to be successful on the basis of anecdotal, qualitative, and quantitative data

Figure 4-4.
PILOT SITE PRE- AND POSTIMPLEMENTATION CHANGE IN TIME FOR SHIFT CHANGE

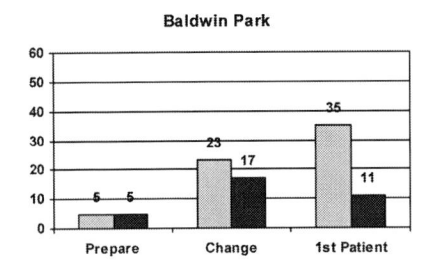

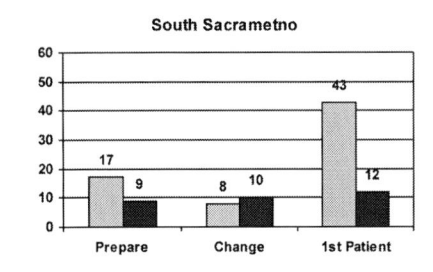

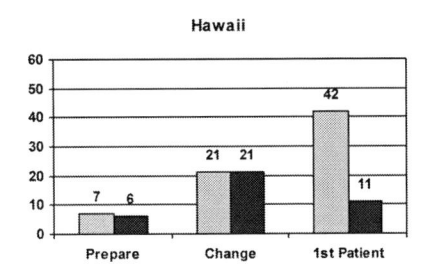

Baldwin Park
- Prepare: 5, 5
- Change: 23, 17
- 1st Patient: 35, 11

South Sacrametno
- Prepare: 17, 9
- Change: 8, 10
- 1st Patient: 43, 12

Hawaii
- Prepare: 7, 6
- Change: 21, 21
- 1st Patient: 42, 11

Prototype / Baseline

Prepare: Time in minutes from arrival on unit to when the nurse receives first patient report out
Change: Time in minutes from the first patient report out to the last patient report out
1st Patient: Time in minutes it takes from arrival on unit until the nurse physically see their first patient

The amount of time (minutes) for pre- and postimplementation shift change at the pilot medical-surgical units at three Kaiser Permanente hospitals is shown. The pre- and postimplementation times were about two months apart. Used with permission.

from the sites. On completion of the pilot phase, we gained nurse executive buy-in to implement this practice in the KP hospitals. In addition, KP's quality and safety leadership, and, ultimately, senior executive leadership through the chief executive officer supported the need to standardize handoffs between nurses at change of shift—and NKE as the practice to spread.

Initially, we intended to spread this practice in medical-surgical care settings in all 31 KP hospitals. However, in preparing for the launch of this effort to the first wave of units, we conducted an assessment of readiness, which was based on leadership engagement and selection of project leads. This assessment indicated that 20 hospitals were ready to spread this practice in all inpatient units and for all nurses—that is, more than 230 care units and 9,100 staff nurses.

Formation of the Collaborative

Given KP's size and status as a regional system, in December 2005, we established a collaborative that would use (1) face-to-face meetings and virtual technology to transfer knowledge about NKE and (2) an accountability infrastructure to provide the content support, sharing of resources knowledge, and management of accountability. As described elsewhere,[5] Web-based audioconferencing was the primary tool used to share learning.

The IHI extranet, a secure section of its Web site, was used as a central platform on which teams could enter data forms to track their measures and post qualitative, narrative descriptions of their work (for example, changes tested, barriers experienced) and share presentations, team storyboards, and other tools they developed. A collaborative listserve was established for administrative communication and to facilitate content discussion. In addition, we provided traditional collaborative support in the form of a kickoff meeting and mid-implementation project lead sharing meetings. Finally, one of the most popular resources was the team coach, who talked monthly via phone for one hour with each hospital's team to help move the project forward and assist in determining how to remove barriers to implementation. Table 4-1 (page 63) outlines the elements of the support system in terms of their frequency and purpose.

We tailored our approach to the respective needs of the KP regions. In Northern California, the medical centers were asked to volunteer for the NKE Collaborative, which accounted for 7 of the 20 hospitals that ended up participating. In Southern California, regional leadership made NKE a regional priority, and all 11 hospitals were enrolled. Hawaii, as an original pilot site (with one hospital in the region), accelerated its implementation, and the Northwest, another original pilot site (also with one hospital), reintroduced the NKE concepts to its staff.

Three-Tier Structure
To support the NKE Collaborative, a three-tier structure was put into place: (1) national team, (2) regional teams, and (3) hospital teams.

National Team. The national team, which consisted of one director, one project lead, three faculty/coaches, and two IHI faculty and advisors, provided all content, coaching, project management, metric tracking, and national leadership.

Regional Teams. The regional teams, each of which was responsible for leadership for one of the four regions, consisted of a regional leader/project lead (who was responsible for communication, reporting progress to the regional executive committee, and coordinating regional face-to-face meetings, along with managing hospital-level leadership issues and needs identified by the national team) and an executive sponsor, who could commit resources, align incentives, and hold hospital-level executives accountable for progress. Day-to-day management and monitoring of the spread project for both regional and national teams was the responsibility of the national project lead.

Hospital Teams. Each hospital team was responsible for the local implementation of NKE, including collection of process data. The teams varied in size from 2 (a hospital lead and project lead) to as many as 10 members, which included every department manager and information technology staff. The project leads were typically nursing leaders of several units, such as service-line administrators, or nurse educators. Nearly all of the 20 hospital teams, on the basis of the recommendations of program offices and IHI that were provided in the set-up for spread, created multidisciplinary oversight teams, which included frontline staff. Four of those teams had an increased probability of more effective, rapid spread of the practice because of the combination of appropriate project lead selection, executive leadership support, and the presence of key staff as part of the oversight team. This was demonstrated by the time it took for the hospital to complete the three-wave process and the reporting and tracking of process measures during implementation.

Communication with the hospital team's project lead and support from the hospital's nurse executive and staff leadership partnering in spread efforts were critical to success. For example, the most rapid spread occurred at South San Francisco and Hawaii/Moanalua, where frontline staff constituted most of the hospital oversight team, the nurse executive supported the effort, and all unit managers participated in monthly coaching calls, regardless of which wave of implementation they were in. The presence of an executive sponsor was a criterion for hospital participation in the spread of NKE. The hospital executive sponsor was responsible for ensuring that all four key success factors listed in Table 4-2 (page 64) were part of the spread plan and acted on.

A Three-Wave Collaborative
Selection of Hospitals and Units. From December 2005 through February 2006, the national team paired up with

Table 4-1.
NATIONAL (PROGRAM) OFFICE RESOURCES PROVIDED FOR THE SPREAD COLLABORATIVE*

Tool	Frequency	Purpose
Kickoff meeting	Once, all day	Unit-based teams, hospital oriented to NKE, improvement methodology, simulation training, and communication and begin action plan
One-on-one coaching for local project leads by trained coach	Monthly call	Skill development, strategy development, and implementation support
Joint project lead calls: open call between national project team and any local hospital project lead	Monthly call	Network and share progress and review of tools and training
Unit-based team calls†	Monthly call	Share progress and overcome barriers
Web-based orientation for hospital-based teams	Once	Orientation: understand roles and first steps
Extranet Web site (Institute for Healthcare Improvement)	Ongoing	Post presentations, tools, and other resources; hospital-level monthly metric sheets; and updates to teams by national project leadership
Listserve open to participants at regional and local levels and moderated by national team.‡	Ongoing	Promote connection among participants to ask and respond to questions
Metrics tools and reports	Monthly review	Monitor progress of implementation

* Used with permission.
† Discontinued after implementation of Wave 1.
‡ Most local nurses did not participate because they lacked e-mail addresses.

each of the four regional teams to conduct a formal kickoff for the NKE Collaborative for each region. The collaborative set up a three-wave schedule for implementation, with two units participating in Wave 1, several units in Wave 2, and all units in Wave 3. Each participating hospital sent its team, and most of the hospitals also included the one or two units that would be implementing NKE in Wave 1. We provided these teams with a diagram demonstrating how the national and local infrastructures should be established and how they could manage spread from pilot unit teams using the three-wave process (Figure 4-5, below). Hospitals were selected to participate in the NKE spread effort on the basis of regional philosophy. The Southern California

Table 4-2.
KEYS TO SUCCESS*

- Strategic engagement of leadership
- Assignment of clear responsibilities
- Comprehensive set-up and planning
- Active, visible support by senior leadership team

Used with permission.

Figure 4-5.
SPREAD IMPLEMENTATION STRUCTURE

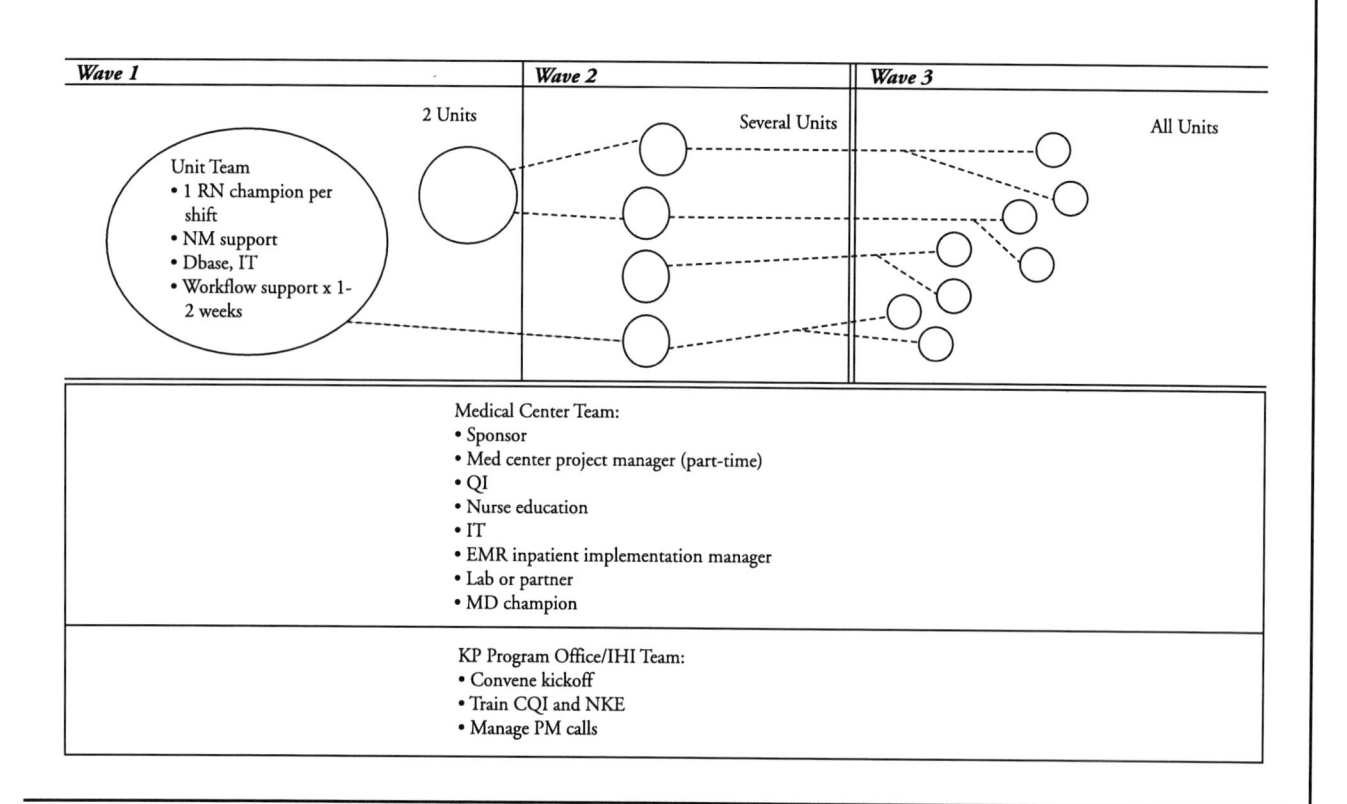

Wave 1 — 2 Units
Unit Team
- 1 RN champion per shift
- NM support
- Dbase, IT
- Workflow support x 1-2 weeks

Wave 2 — Several Units

Wave 3 — All Units

Medical Center Team:
- Sponsor
- Med center project manager (part-time)
- QI
- Nurse education
- IT
- EMR inpatient implementation manager
- Lab or partner
- MD champion

KP Program Office/IHI Team:
- Convene kickoff
- Train CQI and NKE
- Manage PM calls

This graphic was used during kickoff meetings to help project managers understand the infrastructure to support the spread effort and how the three-wave implementation process should be sequenced. RN, registered nurse; NM, nurse manager; IT, information technology; QI, quality improvement; EMR, electronic medical record; MD, physician; KP, Kaiser Permanente; IHI, Institute for Healthcare Improvement; CQI, continuous quality improvement; NKE, Nurse Knowledge Exchange; PM, afternoon. Used with permission.

region decided to implement NKE in every hospital, while Hawaii, Northwest, and Northern California hospitals were selected on the basis of readiness and voluntary participation. Selection of units in each hospital for participation in one of three waves was a local decision but was primarily conducted in terms of complexity science[6] and diffusion theory,[7] and selection was made on the basis of level of readiness. In one case, for Wave 1 implementation, a high-performing unit was paired with a second unit that had turnover issues. These units were contiguous (with a shared hallway), and the hospital's leadership wanted to test whether different methods were necessary for implementation in a "ready" unit as opposed to one that had challenges. As expected, the ready unit's implementation was much more rapid, although the second unit benefited from the peer support that the other unit was able to provide. Units that were not ready needed more time to build a trusting environment, identify key staff and management leaders, and develop overall change management readiness before truly making change in practice.

Timing and Sequence of Waves. Wave 1 generally included one or two units, which would work out the "kinks" of implementation. Three months later, Wave 2 would follow, for which up to five additional units would implement NKE and use Wave 1 units as a resource. Finally, three months after Wave 2's implementation, the remainder of the units would implement NKE in Wave 3. One hospital, KP Los Angeles, implementing waves every three months, used a four-wave system because of the large number of units implementing the practice. Another hospital, KP South San Francisco, implemented NKE only on its five medical-surgical units, with a new wave every month, for completion of all three waves within three months. There was no apparent difference in ability to sustain NKE on the basis of the timing and sequencing of waves.

Support for Hospital Teams

The spread collaborative was constructed to provide the right information at the right time through a variety of tools (Table 4-1).

Education and Training. The primary educational focus was on building skills in the hospital's project leader. The national team developed a 12-month work plan to identify what content should be taught at each stage of implementation—planning, implementation (for each wave), evaluation, and sustainability six months after implementation. The national team and IHI provided training via face-to-face meetings and conference calls, while follow-up monitoring and support of learning were provided via monthly one-on-one coaching calls and the use of the listserve and extranet. For example, use of the Model for Improvement[8] was taught at the very first meeting, and strategies and practices to sustain change were taught via joint calls with the project lead in the final three months of the spread implementation. Monitoring of the application of these skills was provided monthly by the one-on-one coach. Evidence of successful application was demonstrated by a unit's ability to maintain at least 85% of the staff's use of the NKE practices up to six months postimplementation.

Data Collection Support and Tools. Because the outcome data, such as reductions in falls, would not show a systemwide effect for many months, logic modeling[9] was used to derive the process measures that should be tracked. Data on the measures that indicated whether the staff on the units were using the four components of NKE—bedside rounds, patient goal board, previous shift prep, and structured report—were collected monthly. The measures consisted of 14 questions that the oncoming nurse would complete by circling "yes" or "no" after receiving a report for the day. The list of questions is outlined in Table 4-3 (page 66). Data were collected every two weeks during implementation and monthly thereafter for six months after implementation was complete. Measures of success were defined as follows:

- Green light: > 85% of staff responded "yes" to the 14 questions
- Yellow light: 50%–84% of staff responded "yes"
- Red light: < 50% of staff responded "yes"

Interventions were targeted if movement was negative or slower than anticipated. For example, after a few months of data gathering in units across all regions, it was clear that the majority of hospitals were having difficulty implementing bedside rounds. When we asked the local project leads to check in with their teams, using observation and interviews, they found two barriers to implementation. First,

Table 4-3.
PROCESS MEASURE QUESTIONS*

Was the staffing assignment complete before your arrival on shift?
Do you know the name of the nurse who took care of your patients on the previous shift?
Was a patient care information report printed prior to your arrival?
Was the information in the kardex and neuron in agreement at the beginning of the shift?
Is a patient care board available in your room?
Was the plan of care written on the board from the prior shift?
Did shift change happen face-to-face?
Did shift change happen at the bedside?
Did you receive a report in structured format (e.g., iSBAR)?
For patients who could have teach-back, did you do patient teach-back during the oncoming report?
Was the patient's understanding of the plan similar to your plan of care?
Was the goal for plan of care achieved from the previous shift?
Do you plan on giving a shift change report in iSBAR format?

*Kardex refers to Kaiser Permanente's cardex patient record report for nursing; neuron refers to the electronic shift report tool; iSBAR, Identification–Situation–Background–Assessment–Recommendation. Used with permission.

many nurses falsely believed that talking about patient data with the patient at bedside (in a semi-private room) would be a violation of the Health Insurance Portability and Accountability Act (HIPAA). Second, many nurses, having spent so many years performing shift change in conference rooms, were experiencing "stage fright" when required to conduct the shift change in front of an audience (the oncoming nurse and patient).

The KP national, regional, and local teams, working together, tailored interventions to address both of these issues. We worked with local, regional, and national HIPAA officers to reassure nurses that NKE represented good patient care and did not represent a violation as long as nurses followed similar reasonable practices that physicians used when performing bedside rounds, such as pulling the privacy curtain, talking in a low voice, and not providing protected health information on the goal boards. To address the stage fright issue, simulations were conducted using scripted language to allow nurses to practice the skills in a safe environment.

Each hospital posted its unit- and hospital-level process measures on the extranet. Table 4-4 (page 67) and Table 4-5 (page 68) show samples of unit-level and hospital-level reports that were used as "green light" indicators to view how well each unit in a hospital was progressing with implementation of the practice. Every month, the coach reviewed these reports with the hospital project leads. For example, when reviewing the progress in using patient teach-back in Wave 1 units, the project manager could see that nurses on 1-West progressed from 60% using the practice in March 2006 to 100% using it by August 2006. At the same time, the project manager observed that a second unit, 2-West, progressed from 14% to 77% use during the same period. This at-a-glance view of progress enabled each unit to adjust its priorities on the basis of what percentage of staff were using each aspect of the practice. In addition, the project manager could ask a high-performing unit to help a unit that was having difficulty with a specific aspect of the practice.

The coaches and the other members of the national project team reviewed the reports and discussed implementation issues for each hospital. If an issue was identified that involved hospital-level leadership, the issue was referred to

Table 4-4.
SAMPLE OF UNIT-LEVEL TRACKING OF PROCESS MEASURE QUESTIONS*

6 Center Questions	Baseline	Mar-06	Apr-06
Do you know the name of the nurse who took care of your patients on the previous shift?	100%	100%	100%
Was patient care information report ready prior to your arrival?	93%	93%	100%
Was the information on the active orders and on the change of shift report in agreement at the beginning of the shift?	100%	93%	100%
Is a patient care board available in your room?	100%	93%	100%
Was the goal(s) for the day written on the board from the prior shift?	47%	60%	89%
Did shift change happen face-to-face?	100%	100%	100%
Did shift change/walking rounds happen at the bedside?	40%	80%	100%
Did you receive report in structured report format using a shift change tool?	0%	87%	89%
Did you have patient (or parent) teach-back of goals during the shift?	40%	67%	89%
Was the patient's (or parent's) understanding of the goal(s) for the day similar to your goal(s)?	93%	67%	89%
Was the goal for plan of care achieved from the previous shift?	80%	80%	89%
Was discharge planning information on the patient care board?	0%	13%	11%
*How important is the nurse knowledge exchange method of shift report in helping you feel prepared to care for your patients at the beginning of the shift? 4 and 5	0%	53%	44%
Do you plan on giving shift change report in structured report format?	0%	87%	100%

*The questions used for this process monitoring tool varied slightly by region. For the "importance" question we asked project managers to report responses on a Likert scale of 1-5 (1, not at all; 5, extremely). They recorded only 4s and 5s. Light gray denotes green light (≥ 85%), white denotes yellow light (50%-84%), and dark gray denotes red light (< 50%). Used with permission.

the regional team for follow-up. Other issues were directly resolved either via coaching with the project lead or by changing implementation plans at the national level. Some hospitals used the measures to set up friendly competitions among units, while others used them to adjust implementation plans. The measures constituted the most important tool that coaches, project leads, and leaders had to monitor progress and adjust plans.

Changes in Spread Plan
At the national project management level, we made very few changes to the basic structure of the spread plan over time. One change we did make was to eliminate monthly joint team calls after the completion of Wave 1 implementation. These calls were designed to help unit-level teams to interact, share, and learn; however, the calls never became a tool of choice for participants and in fact were seen as "one more meeting." After an analysis using a Web-based survey and review of call agendas and participant lists, we realized that there was significant crossover of material from the project lead calls and the team calls and decided to focus our efforts on the former. Initially, we invited each hospital project lead to attend the team calls and invited the unit managers and staff to participate on team calls so they

Table 4-5.
SAMPLE OF ONE HOSPITAL'S TRACKING OF PROCESS MEASURE QUESTIONS, MARCH 2006 (a) AND AUGUST 2006 (b)*

March 2006 (a)

WAVE	1 1 East	1 1 West	1 2 East	1 2 West	2 3 East-Tele	2 3 West-Tele	2 4East	2 M/B	2 Malama W	3 Malama E	3 Peds
Questions	% Yes	% Yes	% Yes	% Yes	% Yes	% Yes	% Yes	% Yes	% Yes	% Yes	% Yes
Do you know the name of the nurse who took care of your patients on the previous shift?	100%	90%		86%	70%	75%	55%	50%	30%	100%	
Was patient care information report printed prior to your arrival?	67%	80%		86%	100%	92%	55%	83%	30%	29%	
Was the information in the kardex and neuron in agreement at the beginning of the shift?	50%	100%		86%	80%	83%	73%	67%	54%	57%	
Is a patient care board available in your room?	100%	100%		100%	90%	92%	64%	50%	69%	71%	
Was the plan of care written on the board from the prior shift?	75%	100%		43%	30%	33%	27%	17%	8%	14%	
Did shift change happen face-to-face?	100%	100%		100%	100%	92%	27%	0%	15%	57%	
did shift change happen at the bedside?	100%	70%		71%	80%	75%	9%	0%	0%	0%	
Did you receive report in ISBAR format?	42%	70%		86%	50%	67%	55%	0%	0%	0%	
For patients who could have teachback, did you do patient teach-back during the oncoming report?	42%	60%		14%	50%	25%	18%	0%	0%	0%	
Was the patient's understanding of the plan similar to your plan of care?	58%	100%		71%	90%	92%	55%	0%	18%	29%	
Was the goal for plan of care achieved from the previous shift?	67%	80%		71%	70%	92%	45%	17%	31%	0%	
Do you plan on giving shift change report in ISBAR format?	83%	60%		71%	50%	92%	55%	33%	85%	43%	

August 2006 (b)

Component	#	Questions	WAVE 1 1 East	1 1 West	1 2 East	1 2 West	2 3 East-Tele	2 3 West-Tele	2 4East	2 M/B	2 Malama W	3 Malama E	3 Peds
			% Yes	% Yes	% Yes	% Yes	% Yes	% Yes	% Yes	% Yes	% Yes	% Yes	% Yes
SP	1CN	Was the staffing assignment complete before your arrival on shift?	100%	100%	25%	100%	100%	100%	100%	100%	100%	30%	
SP	2CN	Was patient care information printed/prepared before you came on shift?	100%	100%	32%	100%	0%	100%	100%	100%	100%	23%	
SP	1	Do you know the name of the nurse who took care of your patients on the previous shift?	100%	89%	91%	100%	100%	67%	100%	82%	100%	100%	
SP	2	Was patient care information report printed prior to your arrival?	92%	100%	73%	100%	100%	100%	100%	64%	70%	55%	
SP	3	Was the information in the kardex and neuron in agreement at the beginning of the shift?	77%	100%	64%	100%	100%	67%	70%	91%	90%	91%	
G	4	Is a patient care board available in your room?	100%	100%	100%	100%	100%	100%	100%	91%	90%	100%	
G	5	Was the plan of care written on the board from the prior shift?	69%	100%	82%	77%	100%	100%	80%	64%	30%	45%	
B	6	Did shift change happen face-to-face?	100%	100%	100%	100%	100%	100%	100%	100%	100%	100%	
B	7	did shift change happen at the bedside?	92%	67%	73%	85%	88%	67%	29%	82%	90%	73%	
B	8	Did you receive report in ISBAR format?	84%	100%	73%	92%	100%	100%	70%	91%	60%	46%	
B	9	For patients who could have teachback, did you do patient teach-back during the oncoming report?	23%	100%	55%	77%	88%	100%	19%	55%	0%	27%	
B	10	Was the patient's understanding of the plan similar to your plan of care?	100%	100%	100%	92%	100%	100%	49%	91%	60%	82%	
B	11	Was the goal for plan of care achieved from the previous shift?	92%	100%	82%	100%	100%	67%	50%	91%	70%	82%	
B	14	Do you plan on giving shift change report in ISBAR format?	77%	100%	100%	85%	100%	100%	80%	91%	60%	64%	

*The before-and-after view of the spreadsheet was used by project managers to monitor progress across an entire hospital. Moving from left to right, they can view each unit in the three waves and expect that Wave 1 units move to "green light" status before starting the Wave 2 and Wave 3 units. Light gray denotes green light (≥ 85%), white denotes yellow light (50%-84%), and dark gray denotes red light (< 50%). SP, shift preparation; G, goal board; B, bedside round. Used with permission.

could also learn skills and share. In reality, the project leads were the primary participants in both their own project lead monthly calls and the team calls.

Results

Unit- and Hospital-Level Data

Individual units and hospitals have tracked and reported the percentage of nurses consistently using each of NKE's four components—bedside rounds, patient goal board, previous shift prep, and structured report—during implementation and through the "sustainability phase"—six months after implementation on any given unit. Data for the percentages of nurses applying the practices are monitored in a green-light status report, as indicated earlier.

For example, one hospital, Hawaii/Moanalua, using monthly process metrics for each of its NKE units, targeted both unit and hospitalwide interventions. In May 2006, 2-East reported that 33% of its nurses were writing the goals on the goal board. 2-East used these data to communicate with nurses at staff meetings, understand the barriers, and change the system to improve use. By August 2006, the unit was able to increase use of the care board to 88% ("green light"). On the macro level, the measures in the fist quarter of 2006 indicated that all units were having difficulty with teach-back. Because this was the most difficult piece to implement, Hawaii/Moanalua targeted a hospitalwide intervention (all units) to move this measure to green-light status by August 2008 in every unit.

KP is in the process of collecting final data for each unit that has completed implementation.

Overall Implementation

KP engaged 20 of its 31 hospitals in the spread effort. Twelve of the hospitals successfully implemented NKE in all the intended units by December 2006. An additional 8 failed to implement NKE fully in all units by then but had varying levels of progress toward completion, as reflected in their implementation process metric scorecards. The most successful hospitals maintained the pace of implementation within the defined nine-month time line or completed ahead of the time line because of their organizational assessment of readiness or a sense of urgency linked with other initiatives (for example, implementation of KP HealthConnect).

The inability of 8 hospitals to achieve full implementation was due to several factors, primarily leadership and resource issues. Some hospitals had changing or new leadership, primarily at the middle manager level, which prevented the units from fully participating in spread and slowed implementation progress. Other issues included lack of experience among project leads and senior leadership's inability to provide support to enhance their skills with those of others, or the project lead's inability to dedicate sufficient time to manage the spread process, thus slowing progress and competing with other high priorities. Several of these organizations are continuing to slowly implement the practice at a pace that is reasonable, given available resources and unit-level readiness. All hospitals that were not part of the NKE spread effort have since agreed to implement the practice in their inpatient units. They have all begun to plan for implementation, and many are seeking mentoring from peer hospitals that have already implemented NKE.

More than 9,000 nurses and 230 nursing units have implemented the shift change handoff practice known as NKE and have demonstrated evidence of sustained practice for at least two months. As shown in Figure 4-6 (page 70), within three months of implementation 64 units had adopted the practice, and within nine months more than 230 units had participated in spreading the practice and in collecting process measures to monitor the percentage of staff reporting use of the practice.

Discussion

Success Factors

We reviewed successful spread in the 12 hospitals to guide the design of future spread structures, such as skills and time allocation necessary for an effective spread project and the structure of a hospital oversight team and strategies that leaders and teams can use to successfully spread a practice. We learned from other diffusion and spread work, including the IHI Framework for Spread,[10] a meta-analysis of the available literature on spread and diffusion,[11] and KP's own

Figure 4-6.
PERCENTAGE OF NURSES AND UNITS IMPLEMENTING NURSE KNOWLEDGE EXCHANGE (NKE), BY WAVE

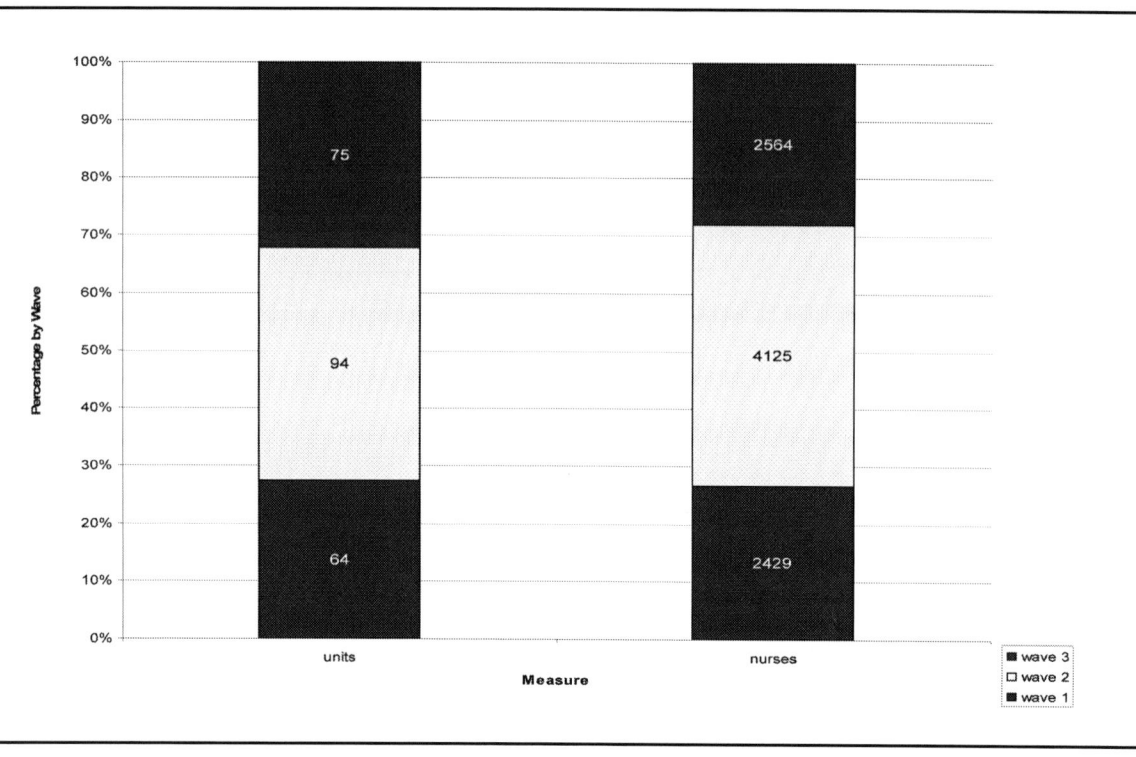

[Stacked bar chart. Units bar: wave 1 = 64, wave 2 = 94, wave 3 = 75. Nurses bar: wave 1 = 2429, wave 2 = 4125, wave 3 = 2564.]

Within three months of implementation 64 units had adopted the practice, and within nine months more than 230 units had participated in spreading the NKE practice. Used with permission.

review of successful diffusion (completed in 2005) to identify success factors for elements of success that may have contributed to this spread initiative. This review identified eight categories, six of which were applicable to our spread work:

1. Change package: what was being spread
2. Social systems and networks in the hospital system
3. Leadership at the executive and project management levels
4. Local system and structure for spread (established in a hospital)
5. National collaborative system
6. Model for spread and sustainability systems

KP folded one of the remaining categories—adopters and adoption—into the social systems. It folded the other category—strength of implementation—into the local system and structure category.

Change Package. The change package—in this case, four practices at shift change called NKE—was, at face value, fairly simple. The benefit was immediately obvious to the nurses, and, once they became comfortable enough with the practice, when talking with patients at shift change, they received immediate positive feedback. A key learning came from the project leads about language and difficulty in implementation. The terms we used, such as *patient teach-back* and *Model for Improvement,* were confusing to staff and presented barriers to learning. Successful project leads simplified the terms, substituting *talk with your patient to set goals* for *patient teach-back,* for example, in response. In future efforts, we will simplify language and coach for behaviors to reduce this barrier.

Social Systems and Networks in the Hospital System. Appropriate access to and understanding of the social system and networks in the hospital system was key to successful spread. It is true that culture is local, and defining how to engage local opinion leaders, define appropriate communication tools, and use staff mentors was unique to each hospital. Several themes, however, were common to all successful sites. Leadership needed to understand who the project lead should be to leverage rapid spread on the basis of that person's role and skills; in the absence of an ideal candidate, leadership should align champions from across the hospital to assist with implementation and use their units as the early pilot sites. Understanding how to use storytelling to engage frontline staff in creating the will to adopt the practice on units in subsequent waves was critical to success, considering the highly person-dependent practice we were implementing. Asking nurses trained in the practice to float to other units, act as mentors and trainers for new units, and simply be present in settings to discuss their experience with others all facilitated spread. One hospital, Hawaii/Moanalua, used "talk story" or a formal storytelling practice, to ready units for adopting NKE and to assist with implementation.

Leadership at the Executive and Project Management Levels. The attention of and modeling by leadership at the executive sponsor level—in this case, the hospital nurse executive—both facilitated successful implementation and helped speed the pace of the spread effort. The more closely this leader focused on selecting the appropriate project lead, assisted in setting goals, and providing dedicated time and mentoring to the effort, the more rapid and successful the implementation. These leaders established hospital-level oversight teams, selected the project lead, and established a process to monitor and report progress. Similarly, the essential aspects of a project lead skill set included social influence, as listed in Table 4-6 (right).

We used the collaborative structure to teach the hospitals' project managers project management and performance improvement skills and coach them in mastering the use of tools and methods to support implementation at the local level. In addition, in February 2006, during the spread effort, four project leads participated in IHI's Breakthrough Series College,[12] which helped them learn how, for example, to develop key technical content, prepare teams

---

Table 4-6.
SKILLS AND EXPECTATIONS FOR PROJECT LEADS*

Leadership
- Have a team orientation
- Set and reinforce expectations
- Empower and respect others

Organization
- Focus attention detail
- Be flexible to customize plans

Communication
- Be open, honest, and constant
- Over-communicate early
- Use public relations effectively

Presentation
- Be clear and articulate
- Be able to create a high-level message about the initiative

Use of Data
- Believe that results drive implementation
- Use data at the unit level to turn doubters into believers
- Help senior leadership monitor progress

Personality
- Be passionate
- Translate learning to implement in other units

*Used with permission.

to participate, support teams during action periods, and spread improvement. During postimplementation evaluation, the project leads indicated that this formal training gave them knowledge and tools such as the ability to understand how to use the Model for Improvement at the frontline during spread efforts and how to use tools to establish team charters and implementation plans to successfully implement the second and third waves of the local spread project. (Only others who had business education demonstrated similar ease with implementation and improvement skills.) When the leads developed tools and plans for their work, they posted them to the extranet so other hospitals could learn from their work and use the tools in implementation.

Local System and Structure for Spread. Successful hospitals established a local spread collaborative that mirrored the system and structure provided at the national level. They held kickoff and mass training events using materials such as educational slide presentations, NKE practice descriptions, and stories and work plans provided by the national program as basic tools that they then enhanced for their own use. One of the most powerful will-building tools provided by the national project team was the retelling of the Josie King story[13] during kickoff meetings. The story of Josie, a young child who died tragically because of multiple errors during her hospitalization, was a powerful motivator for staff, and we acquired the eight-minute video for each hospital to use at each of its kickoff events and for local units to view.

Many say that spread is difficult because it involves repeating what others have done rather than innovating locally. Yet we learned that the hospitals developed and implemented several innovative ideas to overcome barriers to implementation, which produced pride in their local ability to create and make the NKE practice their own. We then asked the hospitals to share their innovations broadly across the system and even with their peers on a national basis. For example, in teach-back, perhaps the most difficult skill in the handoff practice, nurses at shift change discuss goals for the day with the patient. Staff needed to practice this skill, which involves a shift from talking to a patient to talking *with* a patient and asking him or her to state the goal in his or her own words so it could be written on the goal board. Sites developed detailed scripted simulation training (South San Francisco), a videotape demonstrating and teaching the practice (Permanente Baldwin Park), and a media campaign with posters and water-bottle wrappers to help staff use common language with patients (Los Angeles).

National Collaborative System. The KP national project team and IHI provided several support and networking tools for project leads, as the identified change agents, and staff to share learning. During the evaluation process, we used a Web survey of participating staff and a face-to-face meeting with representative teams from some of the successful hospitals. As a result of this process, project leads identified five of these tools as most essential to team success:

- Face-to-face meetings
- Project lead collaborative monthly calls
- One-on-one project lead coaching
- Use of process measures
- Use of the extranet to post tools

For example, project leads used their monthly hour-long coaching time to remove barriers, work through issues, stay on track, and have someone hold them accountable. These calls provided them the opportunity to build their own skills in a customized format. They also appreciated the coach's referring them to other teams that may have overcome similar problems. The calls were also used as a vehicle to support the education provided in the project lead calls. For example, when implementation of a wave was complete, we coached project leads to build systems for sustainability, such as revising practice standards to include the NKE practice in evaluation and orientation and using observation and coaching to support the practice. One hospital, South San Francisco, also included information in the patient admission packet about what to expect from staff at shift change. This helped patients and families become part of the team and support the expectation that all nurses would communicate using NKE.

Process measures were helpful when the project leads understood how to collect and evaluate them. The coach reviewed metrics in every call and identified areas where performance lagged and the team could focus on improvement. Leads used these metrics to report back to the units on progress and help teams practice mindfulness in maintaining the practice. Two barriers identified were the staff's initial lack of understanding and trust in the use of measures and the difficulty in keeping up with collecting data for the measures for up to 15 units in each hospital.

Model for Spread and Sustainability. Hospital project leads and their oversight teams created work plans on the basis of the three-wave approach to implementation, which called for units to go live in sequenced stages, with two pilot units as their model for spread. This was beneficial for several reasons. The hospitals appreciated the opportunity to test the handoff practice on the two units in Wave 1 and build stories of success early and then identify how they would educate and implement other units in subsequent waves. They used Wave 1 to create "super users," or staff who were skilled enough in the practice to teach it and help others solve problems, build success stories, and identify barriers and methods to overcome them. Successful teams used the spread model, adjusting speed of implementation on the basis of the number of units, cultural barriers, and number of specialty units. Table 4-7 (page 74) presents the barriers that the hospitals faced and the strategies they used to overcome them.

Lessons Learned

We have learned several lessons through the process of spreading the NKE practice. Because the KP system has a highly unionized labor force, we learned the importance of creating a partnership with the majority of our labor unions—known as the Labor Management Partnership (LMP)—and engaging the LMP from the very first conversation on this project. In some hospitals and units, when labor partners did not feel fully engaged and it was difficult to implement NKE at the unit level, the team decided to engage labor in a recovery meeting, which necessitated additional planning. The opposite occurred in hospitals where staff representatives participated on the hospital oversight committee. Those organizations were among the ones that were able to achieve more rapid spread of the NKE practice. In these planning conversations, we also learned that the staff was busy providing care and implementing new initiatives. For the spread of NKE to have a high priority among staff, we needed to engage the labor partners from the first discussion about potential spread of this practice. We were able to describe the advantages of the practice from the staff's perspective, given the observation, storytelling, brainstorming, prototyping, and field testing that we had undertaken early on. In addition, we had staff and managers available who could speak to the benefits of the practice and provide mentoring to others who were considering implementation.

Many of the challenges that emerged throughout the spread effort reflected KP's status as a complex system in which local autonomy and labor partnerships are highly valued. KP does not use central mandates to effect change, so we needed to conceptualize NKE as a complex adaptive system[4]—that is, one in which many factors contribute to the success or failure of change. As a result, we believed that will-building, creating a shared vision, and establishing a communication plan before designing and implementing the spread plan would enhance the likelihood of success. We learned that our success was best leveraged by focusing on helping project leads and executives monitor and manage the progress of implementation, such as the percentage of staff using the practice, and barriers to success rather than tasks and time lines. This gave them more flexibility to assess their social system and either speed up or slow down implementation on the basis of readiness to implement.

Conclusions

Implementation of a spread plan at KP required a supportive infrastructure and system to keep projects on track and teach project management training and improvement methods to project leads. We also learned about the need to deepen improvement skills at the clinical director, middle manager, and frontline staff levels. The NKE spread project led to the development of the next phase of our overall quality improvement effort to build improvement capacity at all levels, starting with the frontline staff. Since 2005, we have developed a quality strategy systemwide so that it can improve performance on the basis of dashboard measures. We are working with the LMP and with regional quality and operational leadership to develop and test a performance improvement

Table 4-7.
BARRIERS AND METHODS TO OVERCOME*

Barrier	Strategy to Overcome
Project lead lacks experience	– Educate leads in collaborative management skills (e.g., IHI Breakthrough Series College) – Create hospital-level action team to combine skills
Need for buy-in before implementing or to sustain implementation	– During planning phase and "will building," include labor and management representatives – Use wave model to test implementation in one or two units, generate stories of success, and have staff act as mentors to others – Use Model for Improvement and small tests
Variable staff adoption rate, engaging "late adopters"	– Understand barriers and fears for changing practice, engage doubters early – Focus on early adopters and units with healthier cultures first, and then share learning over time with other units – Slow adoption time line that accounts for cultural issues in units, as needed
When spread is complete, KP HealthConnect needs to identify a single tool for shift change	– Postspread, the KP HealthConnect team convened a session in the simulation hospital and gathered information about essential shift tool elements to redesign a final version
Multiple competing priorities	– Regional and hospital leadership communicated the alignment between the practice at change of shift and fall reduction and patient service goals
Difficulty sustaining gains	– Engage patients and families in expecting the handoff practice by providing information about NKE in patient admission packets – Provide NKE education in new employee orientation – Add practice expectations in employee evaluations – Measure the percentage of nurses using the four steps of NKE once every month when implementation is complete

*IHI, Institute for Healthcare Improvement; NKE, Nurse Knowledge Exchange. Used with permission.

training infrastructure to help leadership, frontline managers, and staff implement and spread additional high-priority initiatives. Our experience with the NKE spread project has enabled us to develop tools and training in effective strategies and structures for spread.

References

1. The Joint Commission: *National Patient Safety Goals.* http://www.jointcommission.org/PatientSafety/NationalPatientSafetyGoals/07_hap_cah_npsgs.htm (accessed Jul. 10, 2007).
2. Personal communication between the author [L.S.] and Douglas Bonacum, M.B.A., Vice President of Safety Management, Kaiser Permanente, Oakland, CA, Nov. 2005.
3. Leonard M., Graham S., Bonacum D.: The human factor: The critical importance of effective teamwork and communication in providing safe care. *Qual Saf Health Care* 13 (Suppl 1):i85–i90, Oct. 2004.
4. Agency for Healthcare Research and Quality: *Surveys and Tools to Enhance Patient-Centered Care.* http://www.cahps.ahrq.gov/default.asp (accessed Jul. 10, 2007).
5. Boushon B., et al.: Using a virtual Breakthrough Series collaborative to improve access in primary care. *Jt Comm J Qual Patient Saf* 32:573–584, Oct. 2006.
6. Plsek P.E., Greenhalgh T.: Complexity science: The challenge of complexity in health care. *BMJ* 323:625–628, Sep. 15, 2001.
7. Rogers E.: *Diffusion of Innovation.* New York: The Free Press, 1962.
8. Langley G.J., et al.: *The Improvement Guide: A Practical Approach to Enhancing Organizational Performance.* San Francisco: Jossey-Bass, 1996.
9. W.K. Kellogg Foundation: *Publication and Resources Overview. Logic Model Development Guide.* http://www.wkkf.org/default.aspx?tabid=101&CID=281&CatID=281&ItemID=2813669&NID=20&LanguageID=0 (accessed Jul. 10, 2007).
10. Massoud M.R., et al.: *A Framework for Spread: From Local Improvement to System-Wide Change.* IHI Innovation Series white paper. Cambridge, MA: Institute for Healthcare Improvement, 2006 (available on http://www.ihi.org).
11. Greenhalgh T., et al.: *How to Spread Good Ideas: A Systematic Review of the Literature on Diffusion, Dissemination and Sustainability of Innovations in Health Service Delivery and Organization.* Report for the National Coordinating Center for NHS Service Delivery and Organization. London: NHS Service Delivery and Organization, Apr. 2004. http://www.sdo.lshtm.ac.uk/files/project/38-final-report.pdf.
12. Institute for Healthcare Improvement: *Spring 2007 Breakthrough Series College.* http://www.ihi.org/IHI/Programs/ProfessionalDevelopment/BreakthroughSeriesCollegeApril2007.htm (accessed Jul. 10, 2007).
13. Josie King Foundation: *The Josie King Story* (DVD). http://www.josieking.org/page.cfm?pageID=56 (accessed Jul. 10, 2007).

Chapter 5
Redesigning Chronic Illness Care in a Public Hospital System

Karen Scott Collins, M.D., M.P.H.
Reba Williams, M.D.

Background and Overview

In October 2003, New York City Health and Hospitals Corporation (HHC) launched its chronic disease collaborative by assembling 15 teams drawn from ambulatory practices across the corporation to begin establishing corporatewide best practices and testing innovations in care delivery at the facilities.

HHC is the public hospital system that serves all of the city's five boroughs. The largest municipal health system in the United States, it is composed of 11 acute care hospitals ranging in size from 400 to 700 beds and providing primary through tertiary specialized services and ambulatory care services, 6 large ambulatory care centers, community clinics, 4 long term care facilities, and 1 home care agency. The system is organized into 7 regional networks, each led by a senior vice president who reports to the president of the corporation. A network typically includes 1 to 3 hospitals, 1 ambulatory care center, and 1 long term care facility. Overall, HHC provides annual services that include approximately five million ambulatory care visits, 200,000 hospital discharges, and one million emergency department visits—to approximately 1.3 million New Yorkers each year. The majority of the patient population has public insurance coverage or is uninsured. (In fiscal year 2006, approximately 450,000 patients were uninsured.) Nearly half of the population served live in communities in which the primary language spoken at home is other than English; at least 12 languages are routinely required across the system. The population is racially and ethnically diverse: with 40% black, 45% Hispanic, 8% Asian, and 8% white. This spread case study focuses on ambulatory care medicine services within the 11 hospitals and the 6 diagnostic and treatment centers.

For many years, the quality assurance (QA) committee of the HHC board of directors, along with corporate and facility executive leadership, has monitored and reviewed corporatewide statistics regarding chronic disease measures. Chronic diseases contribute significantly to death and disability within New York City and are disproportionately present in the minority and low-income communities that HHC serves. The management of these diseases represents a significant challenge to patients and providers alike. Advances in medicine provide many options for treating and reducing the risks and complications of chronic conditions, resulting in improved patient outcomes, reduced hospitalizations, and prolonged life. Yet it has been increasingly apparent that barriers to attaining improved outcomes, such as lack of continuity or standardization of care, inadequate access, and inadequate patient–provider communication were profoundly affecting HHC's ability to provide high-quality patient care and to produce sustainable improved patient outcomes. In 2002 and 2003, HHC initiated a number of systemwide redesign efforts aimed at revitalizing and modernizing its health care system and positioning the corporation as a leader and an innovator in health care delivery. These redesign efforts included capital projects, expanded investment in clinical information systems, and ambulatory care redesign to address waiting time and access to care. The chief executive officer and senior administrative and clinical leadership selected chronic illness care as one of the first clinical areas for systemwide focus.

Launching the Chronic Disease Collaborative

Leadership Group

To develop an operational system that could be spread, in October 2003, HHC launched a corporatewide chronic disease collaborative to redesign its approach to delivering care to patients with chronic illnesses and achieve improved health care outcomes for the patient population. The work during the initial year formed the basis for developing changes in chronic illness care that would be spread across the corporation.

HHC assembled a collaborative leadership group composed of senior leadership, external and internal experts from HHC's Office of Healthcare Quality Improvement and Innovation, the Improving Chronic Illness Care program of the MacColl Institute for Healthcare Innovation, GroupHealth Cooperative (http://www.improvingchroniccare.org), the Institute for Healthcare Improvement (IHI), and HHC facility medical directors. The Chronic Care Model, which synthesizes evidence-based system changes known to improve outcomes, focuses on components—organization of health care, community linkages, self management support, delivery system design, decision support, and information systems—in an effort to improve interactions between providers and patients and, in turn, outcomes.[1] We adapted the health care delivery improvement and chronic disease management principles from the Chronic Care Model, and, in partnership with Edward Wagner, one of its

co-developers, and Improving Chronic Illness Care and IHI staff, we developed change packages for both conditions, which were disseminated to the facilities. As the teams tested new changes, the change packages were regularly updated to include information about the successful changes and the teams that had tested them. Senior leadership at the facilities was challenged to implement innovative methods of chronic disease management in the care of patients with diabetes and heart failure (HF). The IHI experts helped us to adapt the Breakthrough Series collaborative methodology,[2] with the collaborative structured as a short-term learning system that brings together a large number of teams from hospitals or clinics in learning sessions and uses the Model for Improvement[3] to seek improvement in a focused topic area.

The collaborative leadership group, using currently available scientific evidence, set clinical priorities for each condition through consensus meetings and agreed on a measurement strategy, which entailed the corporatewide goals in clinical care listed in Table 5-1 (page 79).

Teams

Each HHC facility was asked to assemble a team to participate in the collaborative. The collaborative director met directly with each facility medical director and other senior leadership to review the collaborative's objectives and criteria for team composition. This guidance was also provided in a prework package. Facility leaders could decide whether their team would focus on diabetes or HF; two hospitals chose to start two teams, one on each condition. For the initial collaborative, 13 of the 17 facilities participated with a team. Of the remaining 4 facilities, 1 facility was participating in IHI's national collaborative on chronic illness care and had sufficient experience to work as a faculty rather than as a new team, and the other three facilities were smaller ambulatory care services that were already participating in a collaborative (on ambulatory care redesign) and could not commit to a second. However, their medical directors were invited to attend learning sessions, and so they were introduced to the work, and these facilities sent teams in subsequent years.

The 13 participating facilities—9 of the 11 hospital-based ambulatory care services and 4 of the 6 ambulatory care

Table 5-1.
DIABETES AND HEART FAILURE GOALS AND TARGETS*

Diabetes
- Decreasing HA1C values to < 7.0 (target, 60%)
- Decreasing fasting LDL to <100 mg/dL (target, 60%)
- Decreasing blood pressure to < 130/80 mmHg (target, 60%)
- Documentation of a self management goal (target, 90%)
- Providing and documenting annual sensory foot exam by monofilament (target, 90%)
- Providing an annual retinal eye exam and appropriate follow-up (target, 90%)
- Screening for depression (target, 80%)

Heart Failure
- Reducing re-admission rates at 30 days after discharge (target, 10%)
- Placing patients without contraindications on an ACEI (target, 90%)
- Placing patients without contraindications on beta-blockers (target, 70%)
- Documenting a self management goal (target, 90%)
- Screening for depression (target, 80%)

* HA1C, glyocosylated hemoglobin; LDL, low-density lipoprotein; ACEI, angiotensin-converting enzyme inhibitor. Used with permission.

---

centers—were represented by 11 diabetes teams and 4 HF teams, whose composition was as follows:

- **Diabetes teams.** Each of the diabetes teams was based in primary care medicine, led by a primary care provider, and included different combinations of an additional provider, nurse, social worker, health educator, patient care associate, and administrator, depending on the clinic's staffing.

- **HF teams.** Each HF team was based in a cardiology/HF clinic, was led by a cardiologist, and included different combinations of a nurse care manager, a social worker, and an administrator, again depending on the clinic's staffing.

The important consideration was for teams to form using the staff available and normally involved in taking care of these patients; this was not to be viewed as a special project in which staff from another area were pulled for a short period of time. Rather, this was the beginning of changing the way that staff provided care. The facilities' medical directors and senior administrators selected the improvement team members on the basis of their clinical expertise, communication skills, leadership abilities, and willingness to participate.

Each team was asked to identify a pilot population of about 100 patients in their organization—a "population of focus"—with diabetes or HF that would be monitored for the collaborative's duration. The diabetes teams' populations of focus ranged from approximately 80 to 120 patients. Identifying the populations for HF was more problematic. Each HF team began with about 40 patients and added to the populations of focus as its processes for identifying patients with HF and for registering them for the HF clinic improved. By the end of year 1, the total pilot population across the 15 teams (including 25 physicians and other clinical staff) numbered 1,178 patients with diabetes and 412 patients with HF.

To monitor its population, each team was expected to implement and maintain a patient database or registry to document the results of its interventions. Software to create this registry was provided to the teams. At the facilities, teams would engage in testing changes and were given dedicated time to work on the initiative. They conducted weekly meetings to discuss barriers encountered in their tests and would then take corrective actions to resolve their issues.

The improvement teams were responsible for working toward improvements to achieve a set of clinical priorities and measurable goals (Table 5-1, previous page). The teams convened for three learning sessions during the course of a one-year period, ending with a fourth, summary session. Between learning sessions, teams were supported through monthly conference calls, written feedback on their monthly reports, and site visits from collaborative staff. Teams were able to report and share results, interact with collaborative faculty, and locate resources through an HHC intranet site developed for the collaborative.

Aim for Spread

Strategy for Reaching the Target Populations

As the collaborative began, the HHC databases identified the overall target populations—more than 45,000 patients with diabetes who were using HHC's primary care services for some or all of their care and approximately 3,400 patients with HF. We recognized early on that working to spread the concepts and changes in care associated with the collaborative would require a multiyear effort. Table 5-2 (page 81) outlines the year-to-year progress in engaging more facilities, teams, and providers and expanding the target population from 2003 to 2006.

The overall aim has been to spread the Chronic Care Model as a framework for redesigning chronic disease care and improving processes of care and clinical outcomes. Because diabetes is a highly prevalent condition in the communities HHC serves and is managed largely in primary care rather than specialty services, the spread efforts have particularly focused on spreading changes that will improve diabetes care and outcomes. However, we have continued to address HF and have added depression. By late 2004, following the collaborative's first year, we adopted the strategy of reaching a greater share of the population regularly seeking care of one or more chronic illnesses. We set an initial incremental target of having each team add one to two more providers (to reach as many as 200 patients per team) and work toward the same clinical goals, as shown in Table 5-1, set for the collaborative and invited additional teams to join, particularly from facilities not in year 1. This led to a total population of focus of more than 2,800 for diabetes and 791 for HF (Table 5-2) and to a total of 46 physicians on improvement teams by fall 2005.

In 2005, we asked each facility (the 11 hospital-based ambulatory care services and the 6 ambulatory care centers) to set the following goals through the end of 2006:

- Increase its registry population to include patient with diabetes who had two or more visits in the past 18 months

- Include the patients' assignment to a care team in the registry

- Improve the clinical goals for the larger population to the level reached with the initial population of focus

In addition, the initial collaborative's goals (Table 5-1) became the corporate goals. We created a network of ambulatory medical directors in early 2005 and began meeting with them; we asked them to take the lead locally in setting specific goals for their service. The new aim statements were posted on the corporate intranet and reviewed by the corporate QI staff, who led the collaborative, during conference calls and meetings with the ambulatory care directors.

Plan for Spread

In planning to reach our aims, we have drawn on IHI's Framework for Spread.[4] Several strategies were implemented to facilitate spread—addressing leadership, presenting better ideas, managing knowledge and measurement, and building social networks to support systemwide change in chronic illness care. We cultivated leadership's active participation in the process. Senior leaders were encouraged to attend learning sessions with their interdisciplinary teams and give

Table 5-2.
NEW YORK CITY HEALTH AND HOSPITALS CORPORATION SPREAD STRATEGY*

Year	Number of Facilities	Number of Teams	Number of Physicians	DM POF	HF POF	Spread Strategies
2003	13	15 Total 11 DM 4 HF	25	1,178	412	• Identify multidisciplinary teams • Set goals for target population • Establish a network for communication • Provide instruction on the model • Engage senior leaders • Establish a registry
2004	16	18 Total 14 DM 4 HF	46	2,890	791	• Encourage teams to work toward goals • Increase the POF • Increase the number of physicians on the teams • Add teams • Corporate build of Web-based registry
2005	17	24 Total 15 DM 5 DEP 4 HF	93	5,043	892	• Continue to expand the POF • Package better ideas • Transition to Web-based registry • Provide ongoing measurement and feedback • Add depression measures • Develop the social network for support locally • Add pediatric teams • Keep senior leadership informed and engaged
2006	17	25 Total 17 DM 4 DEP 4 HF	139	12,470	1,145	• Develop local chronic diseases coordinators • Set systemwide goals • Develop Web-based tool kits • Focus on the corporate registry population

*Teams from facilities participate on a continuous basis from year to year. DM, diabetes mellitus; HF, heart failure; POF, population of focus; DEP, depression. Used with permission.

group and individual presentations about their progress. In addition, we convened two senior leader forums on chronic illness care to address issues identified by individual teams, share strategies, and promote dialogue across the senior leadership. We also packaged and presented better ideas into practical, user-friendly formats for use in the clinics. Decision support tools, which were developed for use by patients and clinicians, were, along with protocols, algorithms, disease-specific progress notes, and self management support tools, incorporated into the electronic medical record (EMR), which is easily accessible by clinicians.

Clinical information systems technology proved to be a critical link in fostering the spread process. Most notably, use of the electronic patient registry gave clinicians the opportunity to provide disease-specific management for their entire population of patients and identify and contact outliers for follow-up care. Medical directors used the data to provide timely feedback to clinicians regarding their performance on the clinical measures.

Teams were encouraged to take every possible opportunity to advertise and promote their work, which they did—by incorporating reports into the agendas of meetings, including medical boards, community advisory boards, and executive and clinic staff meetings. In addition, the learning collaborative formed a social network. We brought together cross-functional teams at the learning sessions and during conference calls and Web sessions that consisted of people at different levels from across the corporation who perform different functions. Teams were able to mitigate the barriers that exist in a hierarchal operational system. During learning sessions, we encouraged teams to actively "steal and share" ideas through table exercises and breakout sessions and storyboard activities and presentations. We noted that even the proximity of the teams at the tables facilitated dialogue and sharing. Teams would make plans to visit other facilities to see interventions that worked well before they began their own implementation. The sharing did not stop at the learning sessions. Team members would go back to the facilities and interact with other staff who may not have attended the collaborative sessions, for example, to arrange follow-up for a patient or obtain some information they needed for a test. The social networks were successful

because we realized that identifying and developing the right change messengers was crucial in operationalizing spread. Spread teams engage every level of staff, from senior vice presidents to housekeeping, in open dialogue around a shared mission of improving patient care. Some network senior vice presidents also highlighted the teams' work by holding "collaborative update" sessions, in which all teams in one network had the chance to report on their progress to local senior leadership.

We now describe in greater detail HHC's implementation of the seven strategies to facilitate spread.

Leadership Support
Since 2003, HHC's senior leadership has clearly remained committed to the organization's goals for chronic illness care, which has helped transform the collaborative's improvement work from a QI initiative into an organizational effort. The leadership supported the QI staff's development and coordination of the collaborative and subsequent spread efforts. The collaborative leadership group, mentioned earlier, was led by the deputy chief medical officer and included two senior QI directors, a project manager, and, critically the chief medical informatics officer. (Given the needed support to make data on the whole population available to the teams.) The HHC chief executive officer and senior vice presidents participate in learning sessions and lead sessions with hospital senior leadership on spreading chronic illness improvements. HHC senior leadership also support ways to incorporate and recognize chronic disease improvement work in different aspects of the organization—for example, nurse recognition awards to nursing leadership on chronic disease teams, clinical information system awards to team members who have worked on the registry, and health plan use of collaborative clinical measures for a pay-for-performance initiative. The QA committee of the HHC board of directors requires quarterly reporting, which includes the same chronic disease measures as the collaborative. This alignment across the organization helps provide the basis for continued work and spread. The leadership's support is also evident in its support for core functions required to support teams—notably the registry, improvement staff, and staff time to participate. Most recently, senior leadership supported the

creation of local chronic disease coordinator positions to manage the implementation of key changes in local clinics and services.

Senior leadership have also advertised the initiative by discussing it with staff at meetings and walkarounds and at senior staff and community board meetings, as well as by addressing it in their monthly newsletters to patients and staff. These are crucial efforts in getting the improvement message out in every possible venue. The improvement message has to be repeated to all audiences and is supported by continually expanding the collaborative goals to include more of the population.

Better Ideas

Specific changes in care that emerged from successful teams during the first year of the collaborative included the following:

- Planned visits to focus on diabetes and HF management issues
- Improved access to clinic visits
- Care management
- Use of the registry
- Self-management support to patients
- Structured follow-up to visits
- Team-based care
- Improved communication among team members
- Decision support

As teams developed and successfully tested tools, protocols, and other resources, we posted these resources on a corporate intranet site dedicated to the chronic disease collaboratives. The intranet site has become a growing resource for HHC—and also contains a password-protected area for teams to post data on run charts and report on their progress.

Information on the most successful changes (in terms of the Chronic Care Model component) from across the teams was collected and summarized for all HHC facilities, along with information on which teams had successfully tested or implemented the change. As this collaborative work developed, the teams and facilities became more comfortable calling on each other for ideas, tools, and other help, which is now contributing to the spread efforts.

Having encouraged all the teams to test many ideas across all components of the Chronic Care Model, one challenge became zeroing in on the ideas and changes that appeared to make the greatest contribution to improving outcomes. We needed to document these ideas in a clear and concise manner so they were readily available to clinical teams and staff and to senior leadership. The following are some of the ways we have done this:

- **Key-change pages.** HHC key changes listed under each component of the Chronic Care Model are based on what most teams were doing and what they identified as contributing to improvement (Table 5-3, page 84, and Table 5-4, page 85).

- **HHC care model.** We created an HHC version of the Chronic Care Model to summarize three to four changes per component of the model that most teams had worked on and found successful (Table 5-5, page 86)

- **Selection of team presentations.** During the final (10th) formal learning session, five teams were selected to give presentations on different components of the Chronic Care Model and the changes they had successfully implemented. These presentations are also posted on the intranet site.

- **Web-based "toolkits."** Tool kits for diabetes and heart failure, with resources organized by Chronic Care Model component, were developed and packaged on the intranet site (Figure 5-1, page 87, and Figure 5-2, page 88).

Communication Plan

Our major approach to communicating goals and practices across the system has hinged on maintaining the structure of the Breakthrough Series collaborative learning sessions and on conducting monthly conference calls or Web-based sessions, producing monthly reports, and coaching the improvement teams. These activities have been the major approach in communicating goals and practices across the system. With each year of work, facility directors were invited to add teams on additional disease conditions and to expand the current teams to reach more patients. We

Table 5-3.
CHRONIC DISEASE COLLABORATIVE: DIABETES

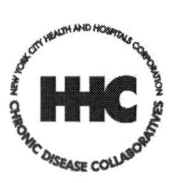

Self Management Support
- Established a model for care planning and problem solving by nurses, social workers, and primary care providers
- Goal setting by nurses, social workers, or providers at each visit
- Follow-up of self management goals by nurses, social workers, or providers via phone call or visit
- Instituted self management guidelines
- Designed and developed self management handouts: action plans, passports, checkbooks, log books
- Education classes and face-to-face counseling for patients and families

Delivery Systems Design
- Planned visits
- Fast-track/mini visits
- Focused clinics: diabetes clinics, HA1C clinic
- Group medical visits
- Designated staff for pre-visit calls and post-visit follow-up
- Link to patient-centered scheduling team (PCS) to reduce "no shows"
- Care management incorporated into team
- Redesign clinic flow to include huddle, goals setting, depression screening (PHQ), monofilament testing, eye exams with camera, smoking cessation counseling, and follow-up (reminder calls)
- Post-visit follow-up by mail or call
- Cross training of staff to perform the necessary job functions
- Regular team meetings to review data, identify areas needing improvement
- Care managers (registered nurses, certified social workers) to do depression follow-up

Decision Support
- Developed and disseminated guidelines, protocols, pathways, visit tracking forms
- Patient education: face to face, groups, classes
- Education of all levels of staff: lectures, in-service, conferences
- Developed diabetes brochures, goal-setting tools, ABCs
- Specialty collaboration with primary care physicians (e.g., cardiology, endocrinology, pharmacy, psychiatry)
- Preventive health record for providers
- Provider chart reviews weekly

Clinical Information Systems
- Registry implemented and updated
- Registry used to follow a population: identify outliers, patients lost to follow-up, track measures
- Reports developed and providers are given feedback
- Diabetes protocol/lab panel/note/summary in Misys
- EMR updated to include diabetes medications, retinal exams, foot exams, PHQ, self management goal-setting tool, care reminders

Community Resources
- Collaborate with HHC Home Care, VNS, VNAB, Telehealth to provide in-home services for patients
- Developed resource lists
- Collaborate in clinical trials (e.g., Treat to Target, DREAM)
- Collaborate with community-based organizations (e.g., NYLAG, Brooklyn Diabetes Task Force)
- Partner with NYC DOHMH
- Establish diabetes education programs
- Developed wellness programs and walking groups for patients
- Participate in community outreach (e.g., health fairs, church activities)

Health Care Organization
- Monthly meetings with senior leaders: SVP, medical director, clinic directors, network team leaders
- Weekly meetings with the clinic chief to discuss progress and provide dedicated time for the meetings and calls
- Regular staff updates at meetings and face to face by clinic directors and ambulatory care directors
- Chronic disease improvement activities reported at regular facility meetings (e.g., quality council, executive management)
- Redeploy and retrain staff to perform the duties required for chronic disease care
- Foster collaboration between departments (e.g., ophthalmology, pharmacy, psychiatry, hypertension clinic) working with the primary care staff
- Discuss chronic disease activities in all facility publications to keep all staff informed (e.g., newsletters, flyers)
- Facilitate scheduling needs

HA1C, glycosylated hemoglobin; PHQ, Patient Health Questionnaire; ABCs, (A1C, blood pressure, and cholesterol); EMR, electronic medical record; VNS, visiting nurse service; VNAB, Visiting Nurses Association of Brooklyn; DREAM, diabetes risk evaluation and management; NYLAG, New York Legal Aid Group; NYC DOHMH, New York City Department of Health and Mental Hygiene; SVP, senior vice president.

By October 2006, there were 12,470 patients in the diabetes registry and 139 physicians associated with diabetes teams. Used with permission.

Table 5-4.
KEY CORPORATEWIDE CHANGES IN HEART FAILURE (HF)*

Self Management Support
- Goal setting and follow-up of self management goals by nurses or providers at each visit
- Self management goals developed with patients at discharge
- Instituted self management guidelines
- Designed and developed self management handouts, action plans, passports, log books
- Education classes and face-to-face counseling for patients and families

Delivery Systems Design
- Planned visits
- Focused HF clinics
- Depression screening during every office visit
- HF fellow evaluates all admissions
- Designated staff for pre-visit calls and post visit follow-up
- Link to patient-centered scheduling team (PCS) to reduce "no shows"
- Care management incorporated into team
- Redesign clinic flow to include huddle, goals setting, depression screening (PHQ), videos in waiting room, 6-minute walks, smoking cessation counseling, and follow-up (reminder calls)
- Use care managers (registered nurses, certified social workers) to do heart failure and depression follow-up

Decision Support
- Developed guidelines, protocols, pathways, assessment tools, log books
- Patient education: face to face, groups, classes
- Education of all levels of staff: lectures, in-service, conferences
- Developed heart failure brochures, goal setting tools, provider alerts
- Specialty collaboration with cardiologist (e.g., psychiatry)

Clinical Information Systems
- Registry implemented and updated
- Registry used to follow a population: identify outliers, patients lost to follow-up, track measures
- Reports developed and providers are given feedback
- Heart failure protocol/lab panel/note/summary in Misys
- EMR updated to include heart failure medications, PHQ, last-visit information, self management goal-setting tool, care reminders, electronic discharge instructions, ejection fraction, and updated guidelines
- Community Resources: Collaborate with HHC Home Care, VNS to provide in-home services for patients
- Developed resource lists
- Collaborate in clinical trials
- Establish Heart Failure Education Programs for South Asian population
- Developed wellness programs and walking groups for patients
- Participate in community outreach (e.g., health fairs, church activities)

Health Care Organization
- Monthly meetings with senior leaders: SVP, medical director, clinic directors, network team leaders
- Regular meetings with the clinic chiefs, ambulatory care directors, and staff to discuss progress and provide dedicated time for the meetings and calls
- Chronic disease improvement activities reported at regular facility meetings (e.g., quality council, executive management)
- Redeploy and retrain staff to perform the duties required for chronic disease care
- Foster collaboration between departments (e.g., psychiatry clinic)
- Discuss chronic disease activities in all facility publications to keep all staff informed (e.g., newsletters, flyers)
- Participate in Medicaid formulary petition
- Facilitate scheduling needs

*PHQ, Patient Health Questionnaire; EMR, electronic medical record; VNS, visiting nurse service. Used with permission.

---

tried to make taking on new teams an annual rather than a monthly event so that time could be scheduled for orienting new staff to the Chronic Care Model and the other improvement methods. Although team participation was not mandated, the HHC president set the expectation to all network senior vice presidents that they should all have teams participate in the collaborative, and as the activity expanded, it became more noticeable to be left out. Encouraging teams to present their work locally and inviting teams to present to board committees, as well as helping teams to present work at external conferences, helped to draw more attention to and interest in the work and promote recognition of staff.

Following the collaborative's initial year, one-day learning sessions were held every three to four months through the end of 2006; we have now moved to an annual chronic disease forum to maintain the corporate focus on chronic illness outcomes. The first forum was held in May 2007. For each session, facilities are encouraged to send new clinical

Table 5-5.
NEW YORK CITY HEALTH AND HOSPITALS CORPORATION (HHC) KEY CHANGES BY CHRONIC CARE MODEL*

HHC Care Model—Key Changes					
CR	SMS	DSD	DS	CIS	HCO
Home care Telehealth Resource list	Action plans Develop SMG tool/checklist/ instruction sheet Follow-up calls and letters to patients Assign staff to set SMGs with patient	Redeploy/ multitask staff Planned visits: 1. Fast track 2. Mini visit 3. Specialty visit 4. Open access sessions Follow-up letters	Treatment protocols Reminders, ticklers, or stamps	Registry on the network server Registry uses: 1. To identify outliers 2. To identify patients lost to follow-up 3. To identify patients for planned/group visits 4. To obtain contact information 5. To generate provider-specific feedback 6. To track clinical measures 7. Clinical ticklers or reminders	1. Provide dedicated collaborative time 2. Educate all staff regarding the collaborative 3. Foster collaboration between departments 4. Redeploy staff to appropriate functions 5. Facilitate scheduling changes

*CR, community resources; SMS, self management support; DSD, delivery systems design; DS, decision support; CIS, clinical information systems; HCO, health care organization; SMG, self management goal. Used with permission.

staff in addition to the improvement teams and senior leadership. The learning sessions have provided a major opportunity to push forward—to assess progress, present data to the whole group, introduce new ideas or plans, and highlight the teams and facilities that have successful practices.
As stated, training materials were developed and made available in multiple forms, including visual and written presentations, pocket guides, and postings on the corporate intranet. These materials were particularly targeted to the key contacts and physician leaders on each chronic disease team so that they could incorporate them in the best way possible into their local schedules, meetings, and other opportunities to work with staff.

Our communication and networking strategy has also included regular meetings with ambulatory care medical directors. This was one of the ways we applied the concept of creating social networks for spread. Our facility ambulatory care medical directors had not been meeting in any regular or structured format with one anther or with corporate office leadership. Therefore, we created a "community of practice" on the basis of their leadership roles in ambulatory care, with monthly meetings or conference calls focused on improving chronic illness care. The meetings and conference calls address various aspects of chronic care improvement and provide the medical directors the opportunity to work with their colleagues at other facilities on common barriers. Barriers have included the use of registry data to discuss provider performance, assignment of staff to multiple tasks, distribution of clinic workload, development of strategies to deal with union issues regarding staff, and medical billing and coding issues for group and scheduled

Figure 5-1.
THE DIABETES TOOLKIT

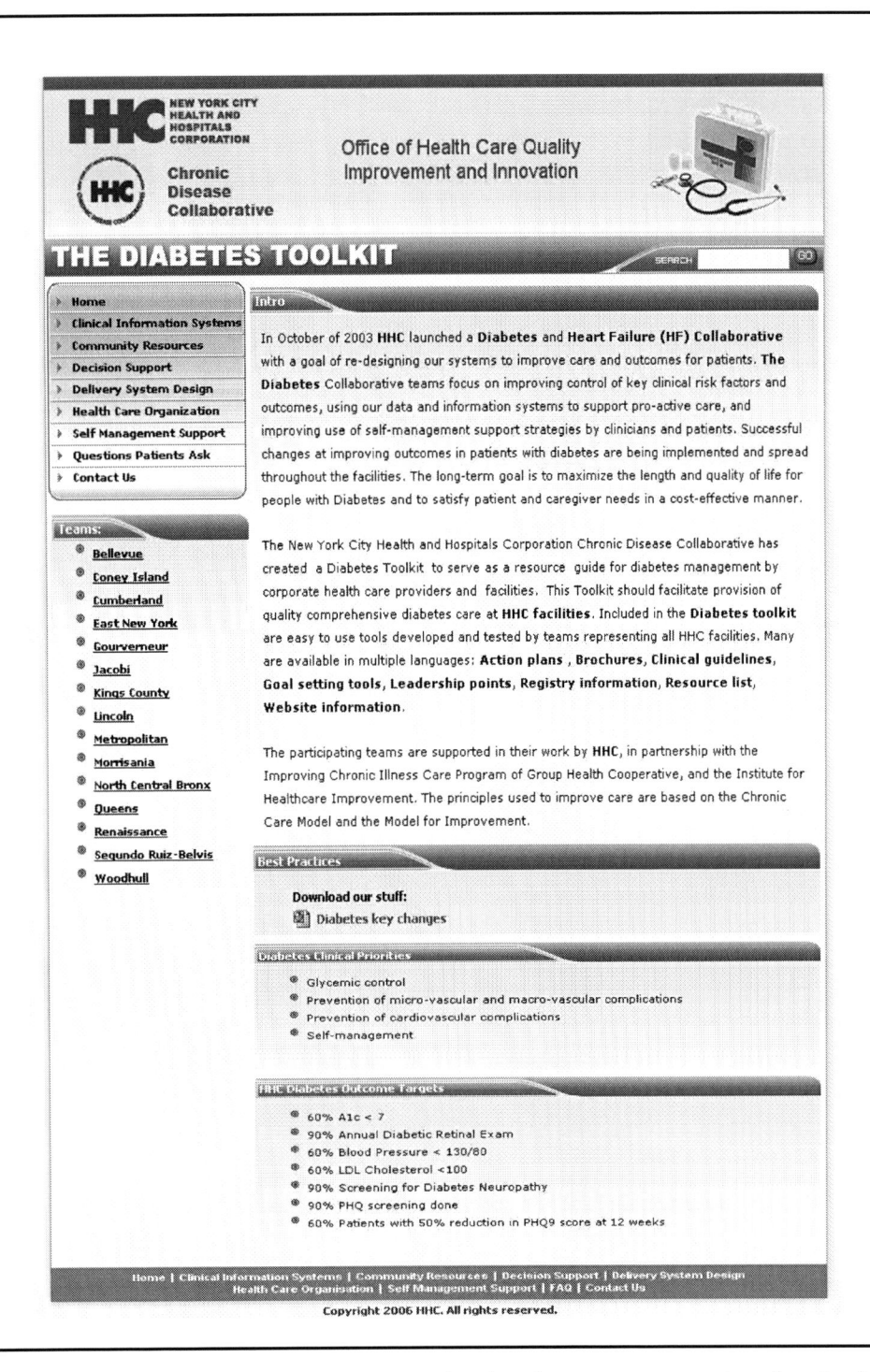

The resources are organized by Chronic Care Model component and packaged on an intranet site. A1c, glycosylated hemoglobin; LDL, low-density lipoprotein; PHQ, Patient Health Questionnaire. Used with permission.

Figure 5-2.
THE HEART FAILURE TOOLKIT

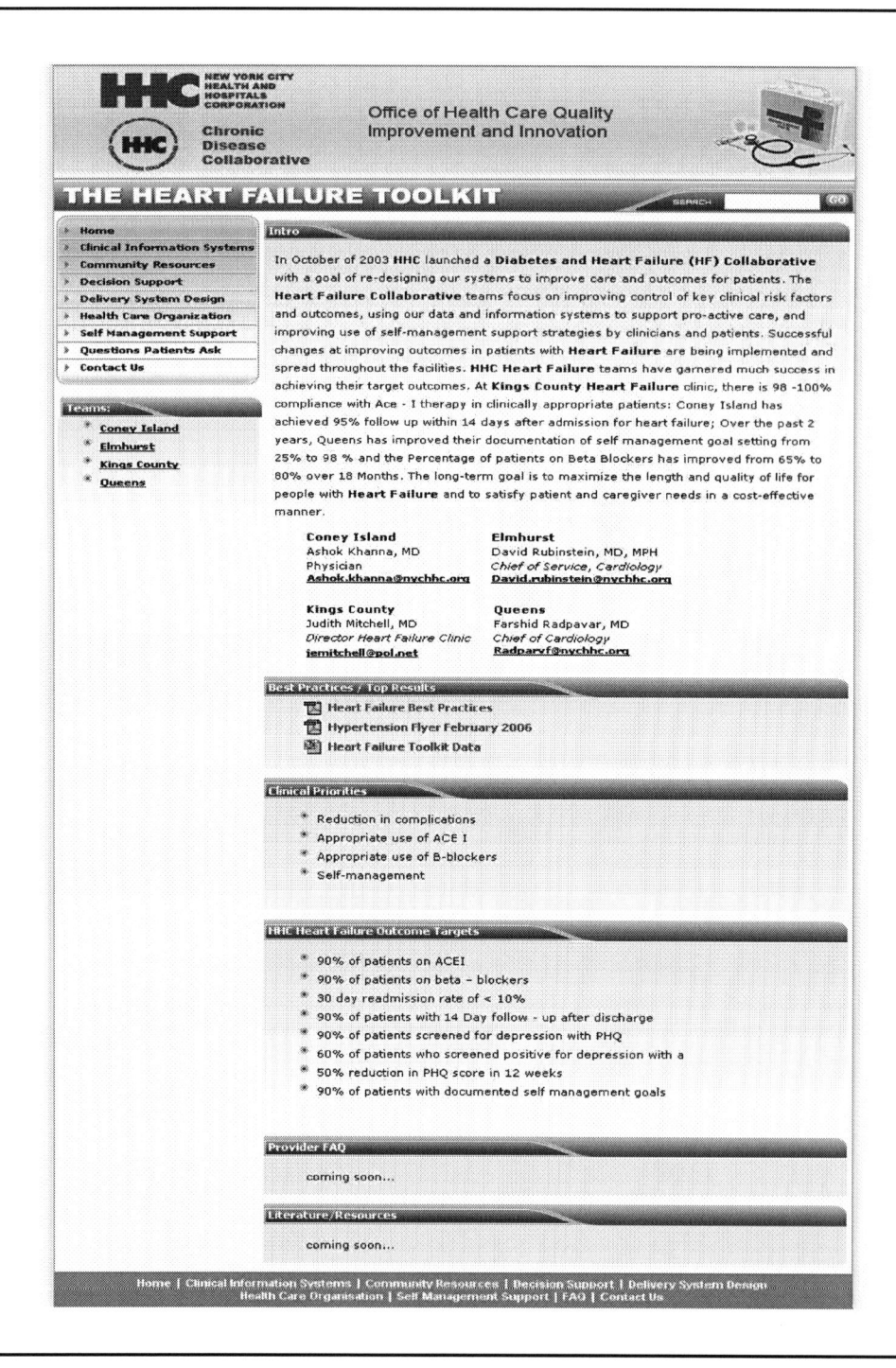

The resources are organized by Chronic Care Model component and packaged on an intranet site. ACEI, angiotensin-converting enzyme inhibitor; PHQ, Patient Health Questionnaire. Used with permission.

visits. As the work progressed, it became necessary to bring together leadership from the corporation's three reporting arms—ambulatory care medicine, nursing, and administration—to tackle staff and workload issues. As discussed earlier, other concepts of building social networks were built into learning session activities. For example, we worked on getting different staff on each team to think about their own discipline and how to craft a brief message on this work to engage their colleagues.

Site visits and meetings at each clinic, in which improvement staff, outside expert faculty, and teams members from different facilities have participated have also been a key aspect of communicating goals and care changes. Primary care staff review clinical measures and targets, discuss facility performance, receive instruction on the Chronic Care Model, and strategize on interventions to improve clinical outcomes. These meetings make it possible to meet with a much larger portion of the clinic staff involved in working on some aspect of chronic illness care than those who are able to attend learning sessions, and the meetings are well received by staff.

Measurement

As measurement has had to address reaching the collaborative's clinical goals in the larger patient population, data collection has evolved from database registries requiring significant manual input into an intranet-accessible corporate registry linked to the EMR, thereby reducing manual data collection and entry. This new registry, which is still in development, currently captures several, but not all, of the clinical measures. In 2005 and 2006, entering patients in the registry was a major activity for the clinics; we tracked the number of patients added to it and compared the data with other system data to estimate how many patients with diabetes were being provided care. We are also able to follow registry use on the basis of the number of on log ons. Increased use of the registry has become one of the newer indicators of the spread.

Through storyboards, we have tracked provider engagement in the process. Storyboards provide demographic data on the number of new clinicians participating and the number of new patients incorporated into the model, as well as details about the changes that the teams tested and implemented. Storyboards are reviewed by teams at the learning sessions and posted on the intranet for their perusal. At learning sessions, they were used to stimulate discussion about successes and challenges. Monthly team reports (senior leader reports) also include information on the addition of new providers and their patients.

The Spread Plan Evolves

We have attempted to maintain a spread process that can be responsive to the teams' and facilities' current progress and needs while entailing specific goals for process and outcomes improvement. We have seen that some aspects of change can take longer and be more consuming than others. For example, in 2005 and 2006, when the teams were preoccupied with building the corporate registry, they were unable to maintain implementation of some of the other interventions.

The most significant change in the spread plan has been that we have had to maintain the collaborative structure for a longer period than we originally planned, but doing so has helped establish an infrastructure for spread. The limitation to this approach is that we have had to move each facility from thinking about one collaborative team and a small population of focus to understanding that *the work of the original team is now everyone's work*. Facilities see pilot projects come and go. Introducing new strategies and goals into a long-standing initiative requires an overhaul of the existing infrastructure, which can be a daunting task. The enormity of the HHC patient population, as compared with the number of patients represented in the tests performed during the improvement cycles in the collaborative's first year, has challenged staff, in terms of staffing, scheduling, access, and work flow issues, as to how to implement the tested improvements as workable solutions for all their patients. Allowing more testing of changes, with larger groups of patients, will help to quell staff's ambivalence about the changes.

Results to Date

The work begun with HHC's chronic disease collaborative has spread rapidly. By October 2006, the HHC collaborative had expanded to 25 teams and included 139 primary

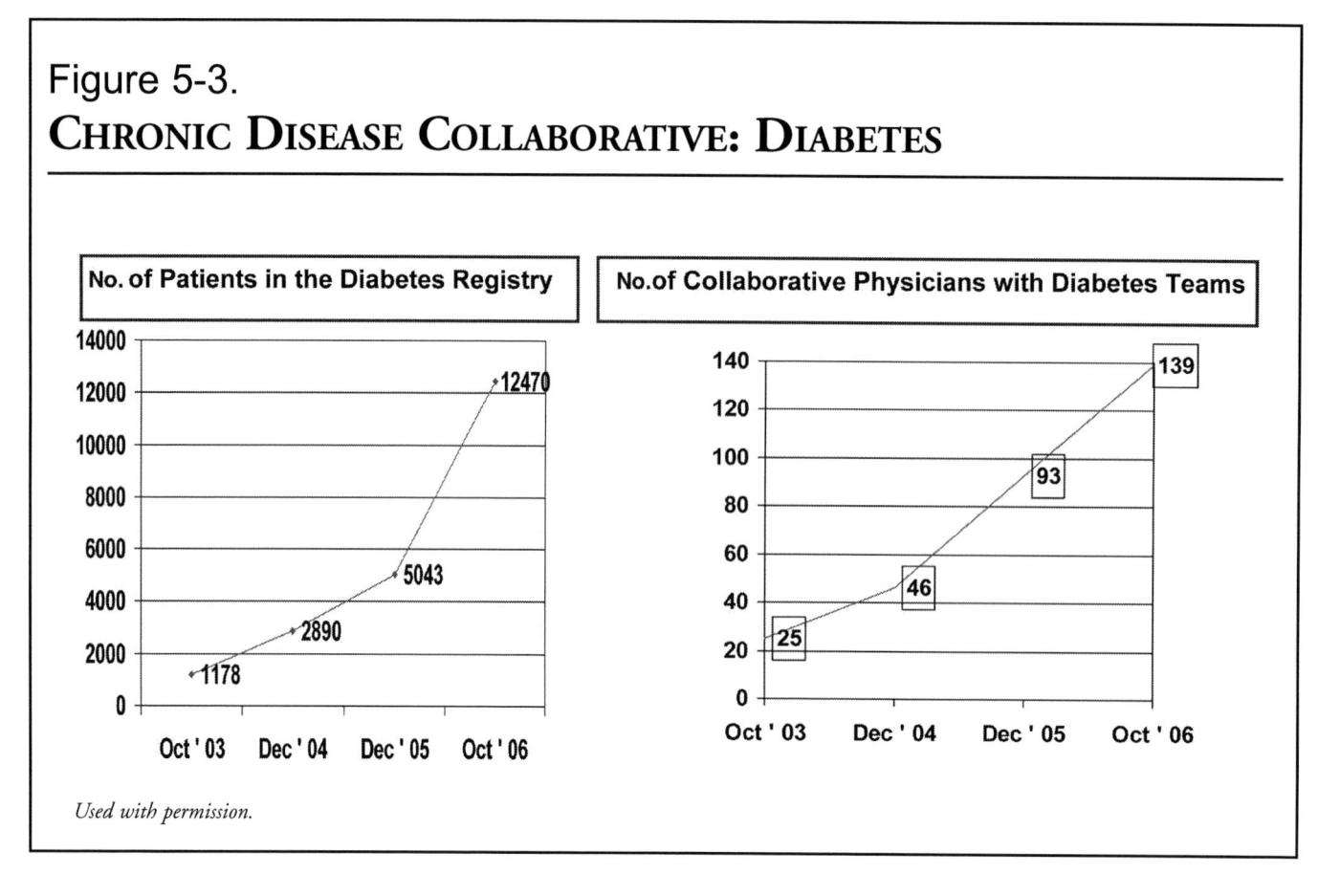

Figure 5-3.
CHRONIC DISEASE COLLABORATIVE: DIABETES

No. of Patients in the Diabetes Registry

- Oct '03: 1178
- Dec '04: 2890
- Dec '05: 5043
- Oct '06: 12470

No. of Collaborative Physicians with Diabetes Teams

- Oct '03: 25
- Dec '04: 46
- Dec '05: 93
- Oct '06: 139

Used with permission.

care physicians (Figure 5-3, above), 30 cardiologists, and 7 psychiatrists serving as liaisons to the primary care teams on depression. The population of focus consisted of almost 12,500 patients with diabetes (Table 5-2, Figure 5-3) and 1,145 patients with HF (Table 5-2) who have been treated at HHC facilities. Although we do not have data on the exact rate of adoption of the changes in diabetes care by physicians in the collaborative, the physicians in the initial teams did adopt most of the changes in the first year.

Diabetes Teams

For the collaborative clinical measures, the documented improvements helped support further spread of this work. Although the size of the population of focus grew over time, improvements in process and outcome measures were maintained. A limitation of the measurement system is that we cannot track results by how long a patient is in the chronic disease program. Therefore, the results shown in Figure 5-4 (page 91) are for the total population of focus for a given year. Our assumption is that patients enter at levels well below what was achieved. This assumption is based on other data sources of overall levels of performance on these measures in the clinics.

By the end of 2006, the results were as follows:

- The percentage of patients with a low-density lipoprotein (LDL) cholesterol level < 100 increased from 35% to 64%, representing an 82% improvement.

- The percentage of patients with a blood pressure reading < 130/80 increased from 31% to 49%, a 58% improvement.

- The percentage of patients with glycosylated hemoglobin (HA1C) < 7 increased from 30% to 41%, a 36% improvement.

- The percentage of patients who have had an annual retinal exam increased from 51% to 61%, and receipt of an annual monofilament exam increased from 12% to 58%.

Figure 5-4.
CHRONIC DISEASE COLLABORATIVE OUTCOMES, 2003–2006

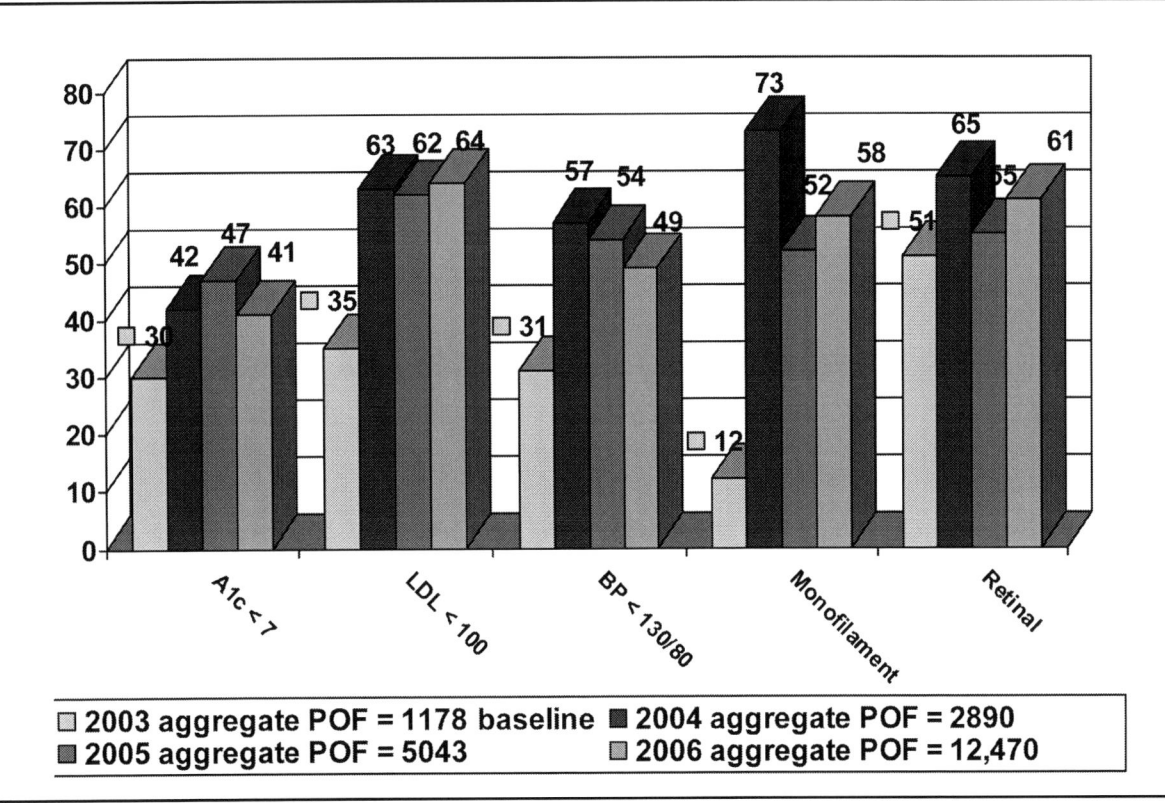

[Bar chart showing values across five measures:
- A1c < 7: 30, 42, 47, 41
- LDL < 100: 35, 63, 62, 64
- BP < 130/80: 31, 57, 54, 49
- Monofilament: 12, 73, 52, 58
- Retinal: 51, 65, 55, 61

Legend:
- 2003 aggregate POF = 1178 baseline
- 2004 aggregate POF = 2890
- 2005 aggregate POF = 5043
- 2006 aggregate POF = 12,470]

Chronic disease collaborative outcomes are shown for glycosylated hemoglobin (A1c), low-density lipoprotein (LDL), blood pressure (BP), and annual monofilament and retinal examinations are shown. POF, population of focus. Used with permission.

HF Teams

The four HF teams participated fully in the collaborative; a fifth team started but did not continue after the first few months because of changes in staffing. In addition to clinical goals, a major goal for these teams was to increase the proper identification of patients with HF and get them into the clinic for the most appropriate care. The four HF teams expanded from an initial population of focus of approximately 412 patients to approximately 1,145 patients actively followed in the registry as of October 2006. The 30-day readmission rate averaged 0%–2%. The appropriate use of angiotensin-converting enzyme (ACE) inhibitor and beta-blockers each averaged 80%–100%, but for some teams, these values were already at those levels at baseline, given the clinics' specialized nature. Three of the four teams also showed improvements in self management support. On average, 80% of the patients across the four teams completed setting of self management goals (versus an initial average of 14%); follow-up within 14 days of hospital discharge increased from 0%–50% to 50%–100% across the four teams; and depression screening increased on average from 34% to 83% for the teams that worked on depression.

Self management plans have proven extremely useful in empowering patients with HF to participate in their care. Patients understand their medicines and how to take them, eat appropriate foods, and make healthy lifestyle choices.

The HF teams have been actively engaging psychiatric liaisons to join them in the clinic to expedite treatment and participate in care management of depression comorbidity, and they have been working with psychiatry to facilitate referrals when needed.

In February 2005, depression screening in primary care was added to the diabetes and HF team goals. This initiative was sparked by the clinical observation that many patients who were having difficulty achieving treatment goals were clinically depressed. To facilitate corporatewide depression screening, HHC developed and implemented an electronic version of the Patient Health Questionnaire-9[5] and the two-item version.[6] Creating the electronic format for the EMR and rolling it out throughout the clinical information systems has enabled us to increase screening and the ability to track screening activity. For example, we screened 53,482 (26%) primary care patients for depression between April 2006 and March 2007—as compared with screening of 1,500 patients by the initial start-up collaborative teams in 2005.

Lessons Learned and Next Steps

Improving clinical processes of care and clinical health outcomes is a long-term endeavor. We have approached this work by continually expanding the number of improvement teams and supporting them to serve as systemwide innovators and leaders of improvement. The collaborative model provided this large system with an improvement infrastructure for ambulatory disease management to enable us to build on and work on additional goals for changes in care. However, teams could not focus on everything at once and needed help in monitoring the implementation of needed changes to improve care. Therefore, the HHC corporate office proposed that each of the seven networks hire a chronic disease coordinator to facilitate progress on the chronic disease initiative (and committed to provide 50% funding for each position). Each coordinator, working directly with the facility's senior leadership and the HHC corporate office, would be charged with ensuring that his or her facility meets the corporate goals by the end of 2008. (Five of the seven networks now have chronic disease coordinators, and the others are in recruitment.) As our communication plans and social networks continue to evolve, we are always attempting to identify key contacts throughout the system for implementation of change. For example, as we began to address depression management, we engaged HHC's departments of psychiatry to create protocols for the overall approach to care.

The clinics continue to need the support of a system that addresses issues they all face, such as ways to provide medications, supplies, and services to patients without health insurance and to work with patients with diverse languages and literacy levels, even while it provides coaching and advice at the local level. Even after three years of work, we are still identifying needs related to aspects of the Chronic Care Model, particularly with respect to self management support and decision support. Our current spread plans include providing more opportunities—through centralized as well as local training and activities—for clinical teams to strengthen their skills. The system-level support will also require more planning regarding strategic and financial resources, reflecting the Chronic Care Model's community linkages, to support a much larger patient population.

Finally, setting clear quantitative goals, as in the aims for spread, and maintaining a focus on data and measurement provides a necessary structure for continuing to move forward. Currently, facility medical directors are using registry data to provide individual- and facility-specific feedback to staff on the chronic disease measures. Efficient measurement and feedback has informed clinicians of their performance, allowed them to review data on their entire population, and facilitated planned interventions for patients. In addition, individual clinicians are increasingly using the registry to monitor the progress of their patients. Their heightened awareness and understanding of the clinical measures and goals and their ability to review their performance with respect to their colleagues promotes improved health care delivery. Facility staff can now engage in meaningful dialogue regarding strategies to enhance patient follow-up, increase patient adherence to the treatment plan, and improve clinical outcomes for the entire population.

The authors acknowledge the significant contributions to this improvement and spread efforts of Louis Capponi, M.D., C.M.I.O. (HHC); Mary Guarneri, R.N. (HHC); Ed Wagner, M.D., M.P.H. (Director, Improving Chronic Illness Program and MacColl Institute for Healthcare Innovation, GroupHealth Cooperative) Michael Hindmarsh, M.A. (ICIC); Marie Schall, M.A.; and every HHC chronic disease improvement team.

References

1. Improving Chronic Illness Care: *The Chronic Care Model.* http://www.improvingchroniccare.org/index.php?p=The_Chronic_Care_Model&s=2 (accessed Jun. 29, 2007).
2. Institute for Healthcare Improvement (IHI): *The Breakthrough Series: IHI's Collaborative Model for Achieving Breakthrough Improvement.* IHI Innovation Series white paper. Cambridge, MA: IHI, 2003 (available on http://www.ihi.org).
3. Langley G.J., et al.: *The Improvement Guide: A Practical Approach to Enhancing Organizational Performance.* San Francisco: Jossey-Bass, 1996.
4. Massoud R., et al.: *A Framework for Spread: From Local Improvement to System-Wide Change.* IHI Innovation Series white paper. Cambridge, MA: Institute for Healthcare Improvement, 2006 (available on http://www.ihi.org).
5. Kroenke K., Spitzer R.L., Williams J.B.: The PHQ-9: Validity of a brief depression severity measure. *J Gen Intern Med* 16:606–613, Sep. 2001.
6. Kroenke K., Spitzer R.L., Williams J.B.: The Patient Health Questionnaire-2: Validity of a two-item depression screener. *Med Care* 41:1284–1292, Nov. 2003.

Chapter 6
Improving Dialysis Care: A Successful National Spread Initiative

Carol Beasley, M.P.P.M.
Vickie J. Peters, M.S.N., M.A.E.D., R.N., C.P.H.Q.
Lawrence Spergel, M.D.

Background and Overview

In 2003, the Centers for Medicare & Medicaid Services (CMS) sponsored the National Vascular Access Improvement Initiative to improve the care of patients undergoing hemodialysis.[1] This initiative was conducted by the 18 End-Stage Renal Disease (ESRD) networks (http://www.esrdnetworks.org) and was supported by a team from the Institute for Healthcare Improvement.

CMS is responsible for providing health insurance for people older than 65 years of age and people of any age with certain disabilities and is also responsible for the ESRD program, which administers and regulates the provision of care (either dialysis or kidney transplant) for patients with permanent kidney failure. As of December 2004, there were 472,099 ESRD patients in the United States, of whom 309,269 received hemodialysis services.[2]

The 18 ESRD networks are private not-for-profit organizations that contract with CMS to provide support to the CMS ESRD program, including improving the care of ESRD patients, assisting ESRD patients and medical care providers, and resolving patient grievances. Each network has a defined geographic area, and together the networks cover the entire United States. As part of their contractual relationship with CMS, the networks pursue specified quality improvement (QI) initiatives. The National Vascular Access Improvement Initiative (which became known as the "Fistula First" initiative[1]) was incorporated into the ESRD networks' three-year contract period extending from July 2003 through June 2006.

Rationale and Aims for Spread

The Challenge
Dialysis is a therapy that cleans the blood of waste products when the kidneys cannot fulfill this function. Hemodialysis treatment requires that the patient's bloodstream, or vascular system, be connected to a dialysis machine by some means of vascular access. There are three major ways to achieve vascular access:

- Native arteriovenous fistula (AVF), whereby a patient's own vein and artery are surgically connected, typically in the forearm, providing a location where the needles, or cannulae, can be placed to connect the patient to the machine

- Synthetic arteriovenous grafts, in which a tube of synthetic material surgically connects a vein to an artery, also typically in the forearm, allowing the placement of cannulae

- Central venous catheters, whereby a synthetic catheter is placed into a major blood vessel leading to the heart

Among those responsible for the care of hemodialysis patients, there is agreement that the preferred type of vascular access is an AVF.[3–6] Compared with catheters and arterial venous grafts, native AVFs show significantly lower rates of complication (such as infection and clotting), longer patency, fewer hospitalizations, lower patient morbidity, and significantly lower costs.[5,7,8]

The desirability of increasing AVF use was reflected in the U.S. Department of Health and Human Services program "Healthy People 2010," which established a goal of 40% AVF prevalence among hemodialysis patients.[9] CMS included this national goal in the contractual expectations of the ESRD networks. The goal was also consistent with the recommendations of the National Kidney Foundation's Kidney Disease Outcomes Quality Initiative (K/DOQI) practice guidelines for vascular access, which has led to a comprehensive set of practice guidelines for a wide range of dialysis care processes, including vascular access.[10]

In the United States, the rate of AVF use reported in 2002 was 32.4% for prevalent patients (Figure 6-1, below). Among the 18 ESRD networks, AVF use varied. As of 2002, the region with the highest AVF prevalence had a rate of

Figure 6-1.
ARTERIOVENOUS FISTULA (AVF) PREVALENCE BY END-STAGE RENAL DISEASE (ESRD) NETWORK, 2002

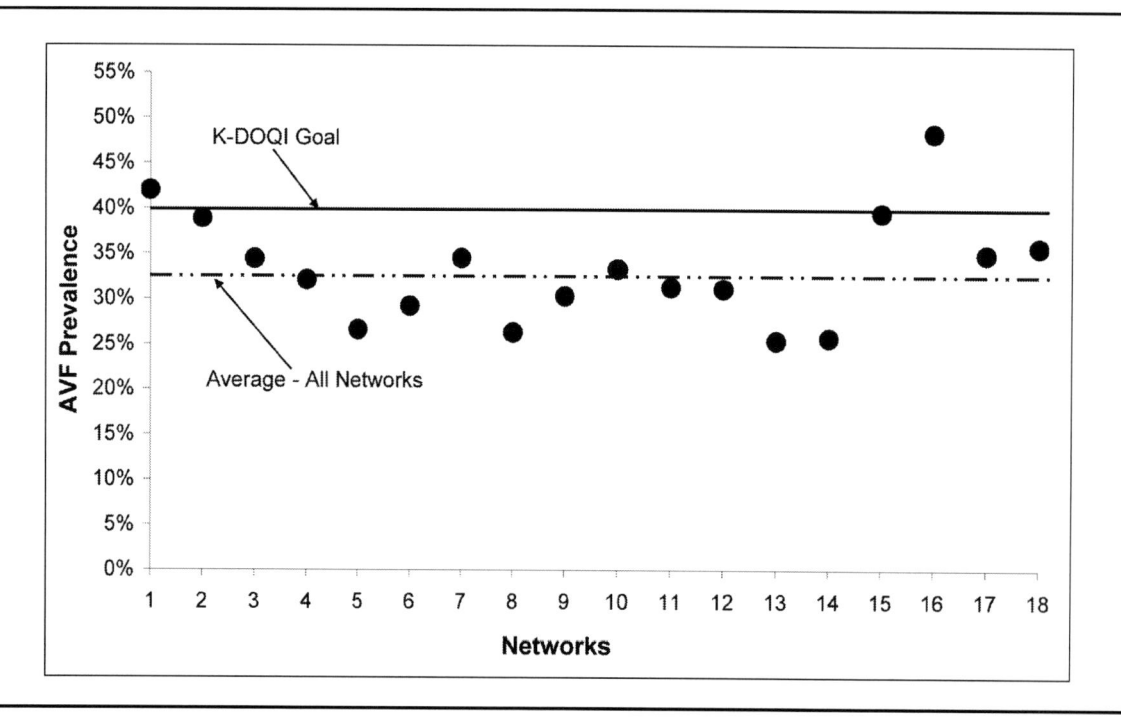

In 2002, among the 18 ESRD networks, AVF use varied across region. **Source:** Fistula First Outcomes Dashboard, *http://www.esource.net/downloads/cds/fistulafirst/fistulafirstdashboard.pdf (accessed Jul. 13, 2007). Used with permission.*

48.3%, whereas the region with the lowest rate showed that AVFs were used for access for 25.4% of the patients.[11]

Globally, there was strong evidence that significantly higher rates of AVF use could be attained on a systemwide basis. At the time the project started, reported AVF rates for prevalent patients were, for example, 90% in Italy, 84% in Germany, 82% in Spain, 77% in France, and 67% in the United Kingdom.[12] Even allowing for differences in the patient mix, it would appear that there has been a significant gap between actual and potential rates of AVF use in the United States.

Overall Project Aim

The aim of the Fistula First initiative was to make significant progress toward the goal that 40% of patients on hemodialysis should use AVF for their treatment. The specific project goal was to reach a 40% national rate of AVF use by June 2006, the end of the three-year ESRD network contract period. The ESRD networks also had individual goals tailored to their specific regions and their starting rates of AVF use. The project had the following related goals:

- Several networks would attain the goal of 40% AVFs for prevalent patients by June 2006.

- Networks with the lowest rates of AVF use would establish "stretch" goals and would make significant progress toward meeting those goals by June 2006.

- All networks would reduce to zero the number of patients with catheters or grafts who have not been appropriately assessed for possible AVF placement.

Change Ideas

Although there was a strong national consensus about increasing AVF use—and detailed guidelines had been disseminated through the K/DOQI initiative—the Fistula First project was the first large-scale attempt to describe how to attain this goal and to provide practical support in doing so.

Change ideas were identified on the basis of published research, one-on-one interviews with a range of experts in the field, and recommendations from participants in an expert meeting held February 25, 2003. Invited experts included representatives from major stakeholder groups such as nephrology, dialysis nursing, interventional radiology, vascular surgery, the dialysis patient community, and dialysis providers, as well as ESRD network representatives. Especially important were representatives from ESRD Network 1, a very high-performing network, and Dr. Vo Nguyen, a nephrologist from Washington state who had reported greater than 90% AVF use among his patients, the highest level of AVF use reported in the United States.[13] The clinical chair of the project, Lawrence Spergel, M.D., also brought significant experience and success in increasing AVF use in local pilot projects in Georgia.

Dr. Spergel guided the development of the "change package," which focused on 11 broad change ideas. Detailed explanations of the change ideas are available on the Web site for the Fistula First project (http://www.fistulafirst.org). The changes are summarized here:

1. Routine continuous QI review of vascular access in dialysis facilities
2. Timely referral of patients with Stage 4 chronic kidney disease to a nephrologist by the primary care physician
3. Early referral of patients to vascular access surgeon for "AVF only" evaluation and timely placement
4. Surgeon selection based on best outcomes, willingness, and ability to provide access services
5. Full range of appropriate surgical approaches to AVF evaluation and placement
6. Secondary AVF placement in patients with arteriovenous grafts
7. AVF placement in patients with catheters where indicated
8. Cannulation training for AV fistulas
9. Monitoring and maintenance to ensure adequate access function
10. Education for caregivers and patients
11. Outcomes feedback to guide practice

Scope of Change

Dialysis services are provided in thousands of facilities across the United States. Some are run by large, corporate dialysis companies, and others are smaller for-profit or not-for-profit organizations that provide service in a community or region. ESRD network staffs are highly familiar with the providers of dialysis services in their regions. However, when the Fistula First project started, ESRD networks and dialysis centers exerted relatively little influence over the kind of vascular access provided for the patients in their regions.

In order to accomplish the aim of the project, the ESRD networks needed to reach beyond dialysis centers to the thousands of nephrologists, vascular access surgeons, primary care physicians and others whose decisions determine what access will be provided for each patient entering dialysis (Figure 6-2, below). This was a major strategic challenge of the project.

Plan for Reaching Project Aim

The project design was built around the Framework for Spread, described in detail in Chapter 1. Spread can be simply defined as "better ideas communicated through a social system." Creating a structure that would allow the ambitious project aim to be fulfilled required the following elements:

- An organizational infrastructure for the project
- Better ideas for increasing the rate of AVF use
- A communication strategy for influencing behavior change
- Strategies to harness the social system linking relevant professional groups
- Measurement and feedback to ensure that changes were leading to the intended outcome

Figure 6-2.
CARE PROVIDERS WHO INFLUENCE USE OF AVFs FOR DIALYSIS PATIENTS

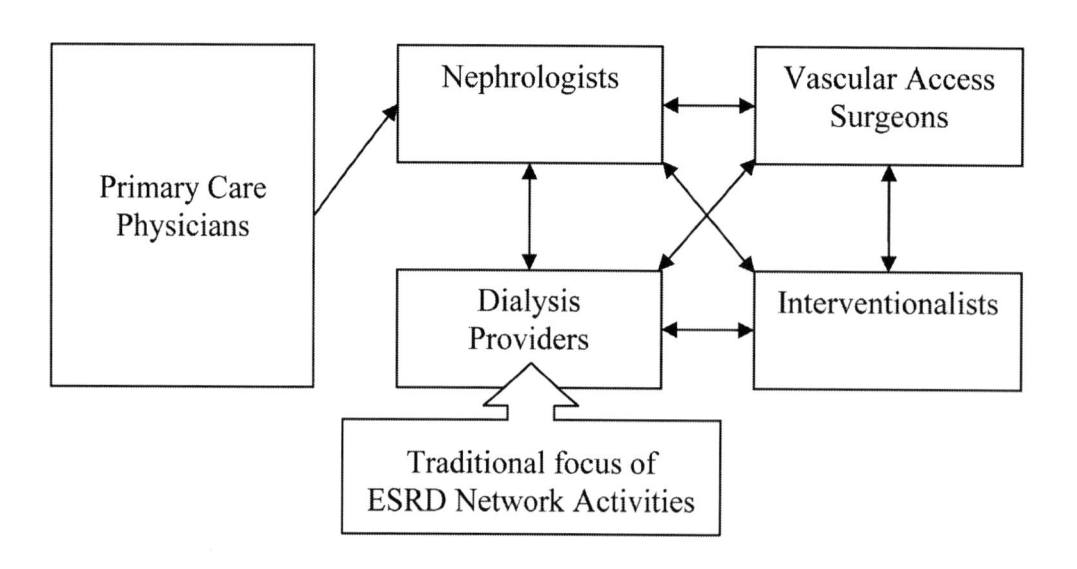

The End-Stage Renal Disease (ESRD) networks needed to reach beyond dialysis centers to influence what access will be provided for each patient entering dialysis. Used with permission.

- Knowledge management to ensure that successful approaches were broadly shared

Organizational Infrastructure

Because this project was national in scope, infrastructure was needed both at the national level and within each participating ESRD network.

Project Coordination Group. A small group with representatives from CMS, Network 18 (the Southern California Renal Disease Council, which functioned as the designated Network Coordinating Center), and IHI was the leadership "hub" of the project, providing orientation to the networks on spread strategy and tactics, setting up regular communication and sharing of experiences and results, leading the design effort for the measurement and data collection process, and ensuring that meetings and conference calls were scheduled and organized and that communication among the National Leadership Group, the Implementation Working Group, and the networks was working smoothly.

National Leadership Group. Representing national stakeholders and opinion leaders committed to the results of the project, this group provided technical input and ensured visibility for the project among all the important professional groups. One important role was to visibly support the change package, bringing credibility to the effort. This group also assisted by bringing the AVF issue onto the agenda of key professional groups at the national level and by providing help in devising coherent national approaches to implementing change.

Implementation Working Group. Composed of the QI directors from the ESRD networks, this group was the "engine" of implementation. The group met in person three to four times per year and participated in conference calls at least once per month. The QI directors were responsible in their respective networks for devising appropriate implementation strategies that addressed their specific opportunities and challenges. The Implementation Working Group members were responsible for executing the strategy, finding partners who could share in the execution, tracking the progress of the project both quantitatively and qualitatively, and sharing implementation knowledge and innovative solutions with the group as a whole.

Network-Level Teams. Within each ESRD network, the QI director was responsible for success at the regional level (Figure 6-3, page 100). The structure of the network-level teams varied, some networks having a team of QI staff and some having one individual supplemented with data support and sometimes a communications or public relations expert. Most networks also had volunteer "medical advisory boards," which were composed of nephrologists, vascular access surgeons, dialysis providers, and patients from the geographic region. Some networks have developed close working relationships with their medical advisory boards and have been able to mobilize them to provide educational and outreach support.

The network-level teams' responsibilities included the following:

- Strategies to reach all sites where dialysis patients receive care

- Strategies to reach key professional groups, such as nephrologists and vascular surgeons

- Technical support to ensure that providers and health care professionals have the knowledge and tools they need to make the changes

- A knowledge management system to document information, progress, issues, and questions as they arise

- A measurement system that monitors progress and provides feedback to providers, the networks, and CMS about progress

All parts of the implementation structure were connected via periodic meetings and conference calls. In addition, the Project Coordination Group and the Implementation Working Group made extensive use of a listserve where ideas and questions could be posted, as well as an extranet, a private Web site where resources could be posted and shared across the project.

Better Ideas

In addition to the clinical recommendations contained in the change package, better ideas included practical knowledge and experience about how to successfully implement the change ideas. One important strategic challenge was bringing appropriate changes to a variety of professional groups. A crosswalk of the changes and the target professional audiences who would implement them makes the complexity of the challenge clear (Table 6-1, page 101).

Once the change package was available, ESRD network QI leaders assessed the readiness of their own providers and medical communities to make the AVF issue a strategic priority. In contrast to prior QI initiatives where network QI directors focused on the dialysis providers with the lowest results, for the Fistula First project, QI directors sought out the centers, nephrologists, and vascular surgeons with the strongest results. Using the prior year's national survey data, the networks were able to develop a reasonably up-to-date view of where "success" stories were occurring. By focusing on success and asking successful practitioners to take teaching and leadership roles in the region, the ESRD networks were able to create a "win–win" dynamic around the Fistula First initiative. Others were then attracted to the work.

Although patients on hemodialysis are the ultimate beneficiaries of the Fistula First initiative, patients were not the initial target for messages in this project. It was accepted that it would be inadvisable to engage patients early in a process and then send them out to advocate for a particular procedure that the health care system could not support. Over time, as the professional support for AVF increased, a stronger patient focus has also been adopted. Now that the system is more supportive of AVFs, it has become more relevant to educate patients about their advantages. The Fistula First Breakthrough Initiative that continues under CMS leadership has developed a distinct patient/family-oriented

Figure 6-3.
FISTULA FIRST NATIONAL IMPLEMENTATION STRUCTURE

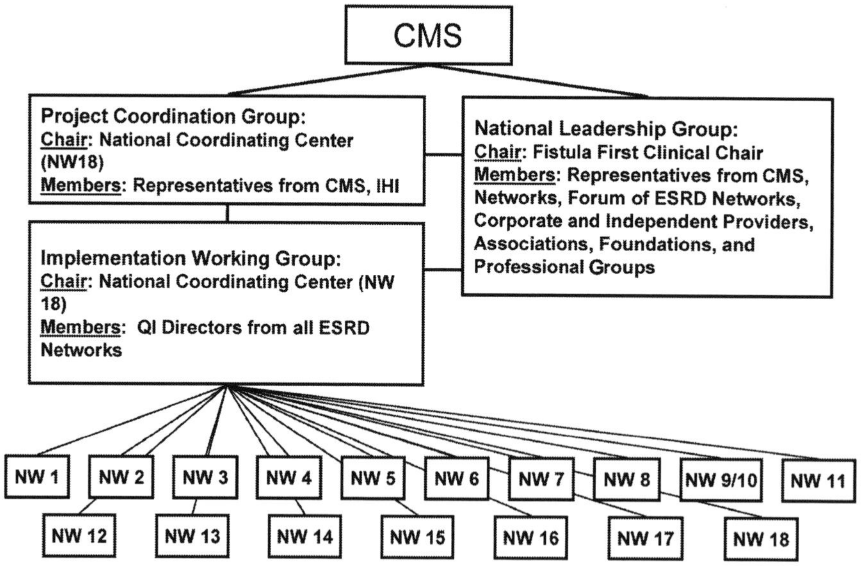

```
                          CMS
           ┌───────────────┴───────────────┐
Project Coordination Group:         National Leadership Group:
Chair: National Coordinating Center Chair: Fistula First Clinical Chair
(NW18)                              Members: Representatives from CMS,
Members: Representatives from CMS, IHI  Networks, Forum of ESRD Networks,
                                    Corporate and Independent Providers,
Implementation Working Group:       Associations, Foundations, and
Chair: National Coordinating Center (NW  Professional Groups
18)
Members: QI Directors from all ESRD
Networks
```

NW 1 | NW 2 | NW 3 | NW 4 | NW 5 | NW 6 | NW 7 | NW 8 | NW 9/10 | NW 11
NW 12 | NW 13 | NW 14 | NW 15 | NW 16 | NW 17 | NW 18

Because this project was national in scope, infrastructure was needed both at the national level and within each participating End-Stage Renal Disease (ESRD) network (NW). CMS, Centers for Medicare & Medicaid Services; IHI, Institute for Healthcare Improvement; QI, quality improvement. Used with permission.

Table 6-1.
PROFESSIONAL GROUPS' REQUIRED ADOPTION OF CHANGE IDEAS*

Change Ideas ▼ / Professionals Adopting Change Ideas ▶	Dialysis Facilities	Nephrologists	Vascular Surgeons	Primary Care MDs	Interventional Radiologists
1. Routine continuous quality improvement review of vascular access in dialysis facilities	●				
2. Timely referral of patients with Stage 4 chronic kidney disease to nephrologists by the primary care physician				●	
3. Early referral of patients to vascular access surgeon for "AVF only" evaluation and timely placement		●			
4. Surgeon selection based on best outcomes, willingness, and ability to provide access services		●			
5. Full range of appropriate surgical approaches to AVF evaluation and placement			●		
6. Secondary AVF placement in patients with arteriovenous grafts	●	●	●		
7. AVF placement in patients with catheters where indicated	●	●	●		
8. Cannulation training for AV fistulas	●				
9. Monitoring and maintenance to ensure adequate access function	●				●
10. Education for caregivers and patients	●	●	●	●	●
11. Outcomes feedback to guide practice	●	●	●		

* AVF, arteriovenous fistula. Used with permission.

task force that takes a more global view of patient education, while some ESRD networks continue to conduct complementary regional patient-focused projects.

Developing an Initial Plan for Spread

The spread effort was intended to reach every site where patients receive dialysis-related care: dialysis facilities; specialty practices, such as nephrology, interventional nephrology, radiology, and vascular surgery; primary care practices; and, in some cases, hospitals. For most networks, the easiest starting point was the dialysis centers. The dialysis organizations were willing to cooperate because it is advantageous to their business when patients don't miss dialysis treatments because of access complications, and AVFs have been shown to have lower rates of complication than other access methods. Dialysis centers interested in encouraging greater use of AVFs among their patients were often willing to reach out to their affiliated nephrologists, vascular surgeons, and radiologists, helping the network QI staff to reach and influence a broader group of key clinicians. ESRD networks also used local chapters of professional societies as an entrée into key clinical groups. Where national dialysis companies had a large share of the market, networks linked their efforts to the corporate dialysis providers' activities.

Each network refined and adapted its strategy over time by identifying high-leverage changes for particular professional groups. Initially, when dealing primarily with dialysis centers, the highest-leverage changes were to institute a formal role for QI oversight of vascular access and to institute cannulation training. Once the reach of the effort expanded more deeply into the nephrology and vascular surgery communities, the networks focused on such issues as AVF referrals, selection of surgeons, and training of surgeons in advanced approaches to AVF construction. Opportunities to develop customized strategies identified by the networks included the following:

- Presence of successful, experienced sites

- Interrelationship among sites, such as geographic clusters or organizational groupings (for example, corporate dialysis providers)

- Availability of effective champions

- Presence of external resources that can be marshaled in support of the project

- Coordination with key social networks, such as regional chapters of professional or renal issue organizations

The teams also classified their spread activities as belonging to one of four distinct "levels" of activity (Table 6-2, above). The levels are ordered on the basis of the degree of behavior change that could be generated, with higher-level activities being more directly focused on behavioral change. Initially, the ESRD networks focused on set-up and general communication (Level 1 activities). Over time, the mix of spread activities became more balanced.

Table 6-2.
LEVELS OF SPREAD ACTIVITIES

Level 1: Set-up and general communication

Level 2: Identification and integration of early adopters

Level 3: Deployment of strategies to get potential adopters to action

Level 4: Use of feedback to monitor and facilitate behavior change and improve outcomes

Examples of higher-level spread activities are as follows:

- Level 2:

  — Network 14 reached out to high-performing dialysis facilities to find out which surgeons were the key to their success.

  — Network 13 identified surgeons and radiologists who were willing to be mentors in various regions within the network service area.

- Level 3:

  — Network 1 worked with the leadership of a large dialysis organization to secure commitment from their top corporate leaders to actively encourage the medical directors of their dialysis centers to reduce catheter use. By measuring, providing feedback, and holding medical directors accountable for rates of catheter use, the dialysis organization focused attention on identifying opportunities to move patients to AVFs.

  — Network 9/10 provided administrative support to regional working groups of dialysis facilities, which came together to share data on AVF use and planned ways to increase it.

— Networks 12 and 18 developed systems whereby staff from high-performing facilities could provide mentoring support to staff in lower-performing facilities to help them improve.

- Level 4:

  — Network 15 developed a spreadsheet tool for facilities to use to track all vascular accesses and the associated physicians. The data were plotted on run charts and shared with physicians.

Communication Strategy

The communication strategy had a number of important elements and was designed to reach multiple stakeholder groups.

Awareness. National and network-level leaders worked together to foster awareness of the Fistula First initiative. The national leaders developed a coordinated set of messages and materials that conveyed the rationale and evidence for the change package recommendations. At the national level, there was value in generating a set of standard communication resources, such as videotapes and standardized slide presentations. Standardized communications were targeted to meet the needs of specific key disciplines, such as nephrologists and vascular access surgeons. At the network level, project leaders considered the available communication channels (for example, workshops, teleconferences, mailings, Web sites and other electronic communication) and made efficient choices. Communications were targeted, when feasible, to the organizations and individuals identified in the initial plan for spread. For example, several networks offered cannulation workshops to their dialysis nurses and technicians, recognizing that not all dialysis centers had enough clinical staff with the appropriate skill to place needles into AVFs.

Technical Knowledge. National and network-level leaders identified key technical knowledge needed to support the project and developed mechanisms to provide that knowledge, including the following:

- *A resource kit to support the initiative.* Together, the Implementation Working Group and the Project Coordination Group assembled a large set of tools, protocols, forms, and journal articles. Most were adapted from existing tools that had been used successfully by one or more clinicians. Gathering the best available tools, formatting them so that they could easily be adapted to a variety of settings, and making them available electronically at no cost enabled clinicians to access practical tools that would help them implement recommended changes. The individual ESRD networks were also able to repackage the resource kit so that it was customized to their region.

- *Outreach to key clinicians.* Successful communication entailed using a variety of methods and messages to spread broad awareness of AVF issues, opportunities for improvement, examples of successful applications, and technical information throughout the system. The dialysis field is complex, with several distinct groups of professionals playing vital roles in the successful care of a dialysis patient. Typically, ESRD network personnel focus on the activities of dialysis centers—where patients receive regular dialysis treatment. However, influencing the rate of AVF use required the development of communication strategies to reach other vital groups.

Stakeholder Groups. Vascular access surgeons were a key audience but one with which the ESRD network staff had relatively little contact and experience. Therefore, the following activities were undertaken:

- Most ESRD networks sponsored special educational sessions (with continuing medical education credits) for vascular access surgeons, where the Fistula First changes were presented.

- Dr. Spergel, the clinical chair of the Fistula First project, is well recognized in the field and spoke at dozens of meetings of vascular access surgeons at both the national and regional levels.

- A detailed educational "roadshow" presentation by Dr. Spergel was expanded to include two colleagues—a vascular surgeon and an interventionalist—and filmed for distribution on a DVD. This activity related to Change Idea 5.

- For nephrologists, another key audience with which the ESRD network staff had limited contact and experience, the majority of ESRD networks sponsored educational meetings, some in conjunction with radiologists and surgeons. Nephrologists and facility medical directors received facility-specific outcome data reports on a regular basis. These activities related to Change Ideas 3, 4, 9, and 11.

- For dialysis facilities, the main point of contact for networks and the distribution points for reaching nephrologists, staff, and patients, the following activities were conducted:

  — Every ESRD network used its existing communication pathways (for example, mailings, newsletters, announcements and presentations at local and regional meetings with both independent facilities and large dialysis organizations) to get initial messages out about Fistula First. These activities supported Change Ideas 1, 6, and 7.

  — The ESRD networks also collaborated and developed a tool kit for distribution to facilities and educators, activities that supported Change Ideas 8 and 10.

  — Facility-related activities included many examples of sharing successful practices from high-AVF facilities and other early adopters through regional meetings, mentoring sessions, conference calls, and other collaborative activities.

Social System

Facilities, networks, and medical specialists are linked to each other through a complex structure of relationships, both professional and personal. The Fistula First project recognized the importance of these relationships and used them to foster change and improvement, as in the following examples:

- Identifying experts within each region who could best teach their peers about increasing AVFs

- Building connections among networks, dialysis providers, medical professionals, and other stakeholders so that they could learn from one another

- Recognizing and acknowledging existing motivations and incentives among providers and medical professionals that would either support or undermine the implementation of changes

ESRD networks used the following activities to encourage key stakeholders to adopt the Fistula First change ideas:

- Newsletters and mailings to key professional groups with information and examples of the successful implementation of change ideas

- Conference calls and meetings (collaboratives) set up to discuss successes and barriers and to provide practical training

- Encouragment of other professional groups to present Fistula First and other vascular access and AVF-related topics at the national conferences of various clinical specialty groups (for example, American Society of Nephrology, American College of Surgeons, American Nephrology Nurses Association)

- Self-organization of groups of "vascular access clubs" in some geographic areas (for example, southern California), to which the networks offered support

- Large dialysis organizations' set-up of their own internal vascular access staff and training programs to support the Fistula First initiative with the help of the networks

- Training by the networks of a group of clinical "coaches," or champions, clinicians in the networks who were willing to work with and mentor their peers on key technical aspects of successful AVF placement and use

Measurement and Feedback System

A measurement strategy was designed as part of the Fistula First initiative. The national project leaders, with input from network QI and data experts, and with the active cooperation of CMS and the large dialysis organizations, created a process for collecting and analyzing data that minimized complexity and burden on facilities and networks whenever possible. Before the establishment of

Fistula First, data on vascular access were collected once per year. By working together, CMS, the networks, and dialysis organizations were able to collect monthly data for the vast majority of dialysis patients in the United States. These data provided an up-to-date view of vascular access outcomes, allowing rapid feedback to the improvement effort.

In 2005, the networks and CMS information technology contractors created a surgeon-specific report on the basis of national surgical billing/claims data provided with the assistance of the Quality Improvement Organizations. Each network received data pertaining to surgeons in the same region and prepared and sent reports to them. The data set was far from perfect, but surgeon feedback confirmed that it served the purpose of creating awareness in the surgical community that (a) this project was important and (b) data were being collected and outcomes were noticed.

An important limitation to the data obtained by the project was lack of process information. Had it been obtainable, it might have allowed a better understanding of the impact of certain change ideas, such as the placement of "secondary" AVFs to replace a graft or a catheter or the functionality of AVFs after placement.

Because of resource issues and administrative restrictions, the outcome data provided to the project were in aggregate form. No patient-specific data were collected, even at the ESRD network level. This makes further evaluation of the success or limitations of the Fistula First project difficult.

Knowledge Management System

To succeed in this project, networks needed to develop efficient and effective ways to share their knowledge. It was important to establish clear responsibility for the administrative, technical, and content review tasks related to knowledge management. A project coordinator (located in the Network Coordinating Center) was charged with collecting tools and resources from networks and making them available across the system. A Web site dedicated to Fistula First has proven to be very useful in collecting and disseminating information. Another easy way to distribute tools is on CD so that facilities and medical professionals can easily adapt the tools to their own use. The CD/DVD training program for surgeons has been a sought-after educational resource, and a similar program for dialysis staff on cannulation techniques is under development. The cannulation program will also include samples of tools, policies, algorithms, and documentation forms.

The Implementation Working Group has continued to hold quarterly conference calls with the national project coordinator; these calls capture the key "learnings" from the group so that these, too, can be incorporated into the change package and Web site.

Evolution of Spread Activities and Spread Plan

Spread Activities

Over time, the network activities and target groups have changed. In 2004, more general awareness and communication strategies were employed, and networks with the lowest AVF rates began working with their surgeon population earlier than others. As the project evolved, more emphasis was placed on chronic kidney disease (CKD) and reduction of catheter usage. The networks still focused on facility-based activities, but more data were provided on catheter usage, and outreach was conducted to other non-renal groups in the community (for example, patient organizations, hospital Quality Improvement Organizations, state survey agencies).

The levels of activities, as defined by spread theory, were consistent over time primarily because the Level 1 activities (general communication) originally directed to dialysis centers and renal organizations are now being directed to new audiences, with more interaction with patients with CKD. Level 2 and 3 activities (finding adopters and getting them to action) are still a significant part of the network activity spectrum but now are focused more on the "late adopters." Different strategies—less general information and more emphasis on data and consequences—are employed for this group. Table 6-3 (page 106) shows the change in emphasis from surgeons to other CKD-related audiences.

Spread Plan

By late 2004, there were signs of progress toward meeting the project goal. At that time, CMS was in the process of designating a small number of national breakthrough

Table 6-3.
NUMBERS OF ACTIVITIES UNDERTAKEN BY NETWORKS TO REACH TARGET AUDIENCES*

Target Audience	Numbers of Activities (Example Quarter)		
	2004 (Qtr 4)	2005 (Qtr 2)	2006 (Qtr 4)
Vascular surgeons	19	15	5
Nephrologists	5	7	3
Dialysis facilities	46	47	37
Patients	3	3	1
Others (QIO, HMO, SA, PCP)	7	5	18

*QIO, Quality Improvement Organization; HMO, health maintenance organization; SA, state agency responsible for certification of dialysis facilities and hospitals; PCP, primary care physician. Used with permission.

initiatives—projects that focused on important priorities for the agency—that demonstrated robust approaches to improvement and that were positioned to create truly breakthrough results with some extra support and resources from CMS.

The spread methodology employed in the Fistula First project had produced excellent early results, so it was formally adopted and presented as the "CMS Fistula First Breakthrough Initiative" in March 2005. In addition to ESRD networks, a variety of other renal stakeholders were invited to join and to provide expertise and resources, as available, on a voluntary basis. Groups representing practitioners, patients, provider organizations, professional associations, and other government organizations took seats at the table, and many have actively participated in the six task forces (working groups) that emerged in response to discussions of relevant issues.

- **Community (formerly Beneficiary) Education.** This task force focused on empowering patients and families through education in vascular access, particularly on promoting materials with a distinct pro-AVF vision. In September 2006, it produced an electronic notebook format of materials for the Fistula First Web site, which is currently the most downloaded product.

- **Practitioner Education.** This task force focused on education for professional and clinical staff. In addition to promoting the surgical video series from the original National Vascular Access Improvement Initiative project, this group developed a cannulation training program for dialysis staff which will be distributed nationwide on completion. This group has taken over the functions of the original project's "Tools and Resources" committee.

- **Clinical Practice.** This task force focused on promoting positive clinical treatment patterns through peer-to-peer contact and education. This work group assisted CMS and the networks with the 2005 surgeon claims data project, developed a list of permanent vascular access codes relevant to hemodialysis, and collaborated with a vascular ultrasound organization on quality recommendation statements.

- **Program Operations.** This task force focused on developing recommendations to CMS and other payers and renal business stakeholders related to eligibility, coverage, benefit design, payment, and medical management strategies. In conjunction with the entire coalition, this group developed a position paper on pay-for-performance in renal vascular access and a list of key recommendations for driving improvement.

- **Quality Measurement and Information.** This task force focused on recommendations to CMS and other renal stakeholders on key areas where significant gain can be achieved through measurement. This work group categorized all available vascular access measures, and serves as an expert measurement advisory team to the clinical practice task force and the coalition. It has expanded on the issues originally covered by the National Vascular Access Improvement Initiative data committee.

- **Marketing and Communications.** This task force's mission is focused on providing support to the initiative through effective communication of messages to target audiences. Three subcommittees are currently at work to update the Fistula First Web site, develop a formal marketing packet of information for consumers and professionals, and refine a marketing plan to distribute vascular access information to a wider audience. This group also existed under the National Vascular Access Improvement Initiative but has expanded membership in its present format.

The ESRD networks continue their work at the regional level in support of this initiative. As stated earlier, now that the "early adopters" have helped to generate significant progress on increasing AVF rates, the networks are promoting strategies that address concerns of "late adopters."

Results to Date

From 1998 to 2002, the national AVF prevalence rate was based on annual data collection by the Centers for Disease Control (CDC) of nearly the entire population (> 250,000) of hemodialysis patients. The annual collection of data by the CDC was deemed too infrequent and nonspecific to provide timely and specific feedback for improvement to medical specialists and dialysis facilities. Starting in September 2003, a system was developed for the Fistula First project to collect and compile monthly, standardized access data. These data, known as the "Dashboard,"[11] are collected both from facilities owned by large corporate dialysis organizations and from independent facilities. As of 2007, more than 98% of all dialysis facilities in the United States report data through this system.

A summary of overall changes in the AVF rate is provided in Figure 6-4 (page 108). From 1998 through 2003, the AVF prevalence rate for hemodialysis patients increased from 22.8% to 34.2%. The 1998–2003 average increase was 1.9 percentage points per year (standard deviation, 0.31). After the initiation of Fistula First in 2003, the AVF prevalence rate increased 3.2 percentage points in 2004, to 37.4%; in 2005 the rate increased 3.7 percentage points, to 41.1%. The average increase for 2004 and 2005 was 3.45%, indicating a statistically significant acceleration over the historical growth rate of 1.9% ($p > .01$). The original target goal of 40% AVF use by June 2006 was attained 10 months early, in August 2005. We know of no other factors that could have directly contributed to this accelerated rate of improvement other than the activities associated with the Fistula First project.

According to network reports, since implementation of Fistula First, the majority of dialysis facilities have designated vascular access coordinators to track data on patient status and referrals at the facility level, a key element of Change Idea 1. Networks have also reported on the major change ideas that proved to be the most significant for driving change in their regions—early referral to surgeons (Change Idea 3), surgeon selection based on outcome (4), replacement of catheters and grafts with AVF (6 and 7), education for patients and staff (10), and data feedback to practitioners (11). The change ideas have proven to be a primary information/education tool underlying the success of this project.

Although the mix of change ideas employed varied somewhat across networks, every network experienced improvement during the course of the initiative (Figure 6-5, page 109). Improvement ranged from 8.1 to 18.4 percentage

Figure 6-4.
YEARLY INCREASES IN AVF PREVALENCE, 1997–2005

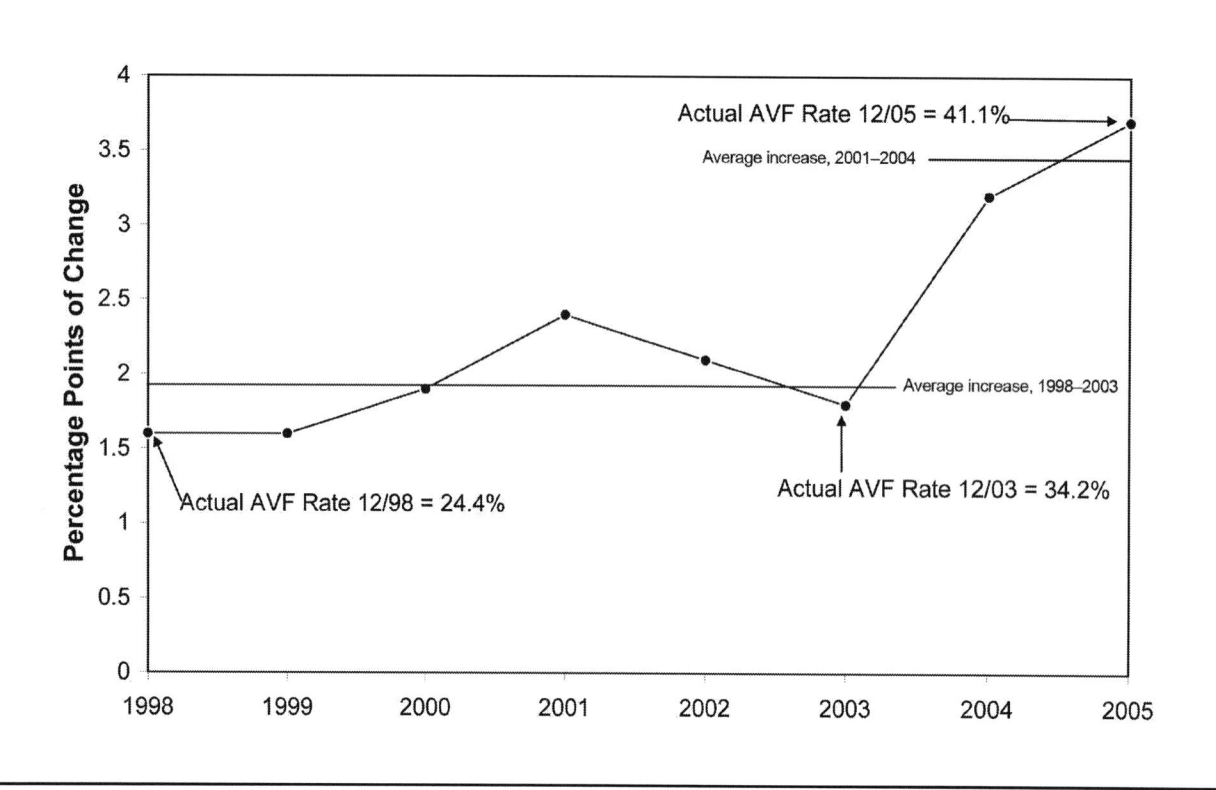

The average increase for 2004 and 2005 in arteriovenous fistula (AVF) prevalence was 3.45 percentage points, indicating a statistically significant acceleration over the historical average increase of 1.9 percentage points ($p > .01$). Used with permission.

points, with the majority of networks showing improvement between 10 and 14 percentage points. Even the networks that started the Fistula First initiative with AVF rates > 40% improved their performance. Network 16 (Oregon, Washington, Idaho, Montana, and Alaska) increased 12.3 points, from 48.3% to 60.6%. Network 1 (New England) increased 8.1 points, from 42% to 50.1%.

Lessons Learned and Next Steps

The major lesson of the Fistula First initiative was that large-scale national spread efforts could succeed, despite the scale of the challenge, the complexity of the behaviors being changed, and the variety of professional groups involved. Few spread projects have been able to show such significant measurable national results within such a short time.

Some factors that the project team believes were most important are now described.

Use of Existing Organizational Structures and Capabilities

The ESRD networks are well-established organizations with experienced QI staff. Although the QI directors in the networks were not equally familiar with the theory of spread and how to develop and execute strategies for spread, it was advantageous that these staff members had

Figure 6-5.
CHANGE IN END-STAGE RENAL DISEASE (ESRD) NETWORK RESULTS, DECEMBER 2002–DECEMBER 2006

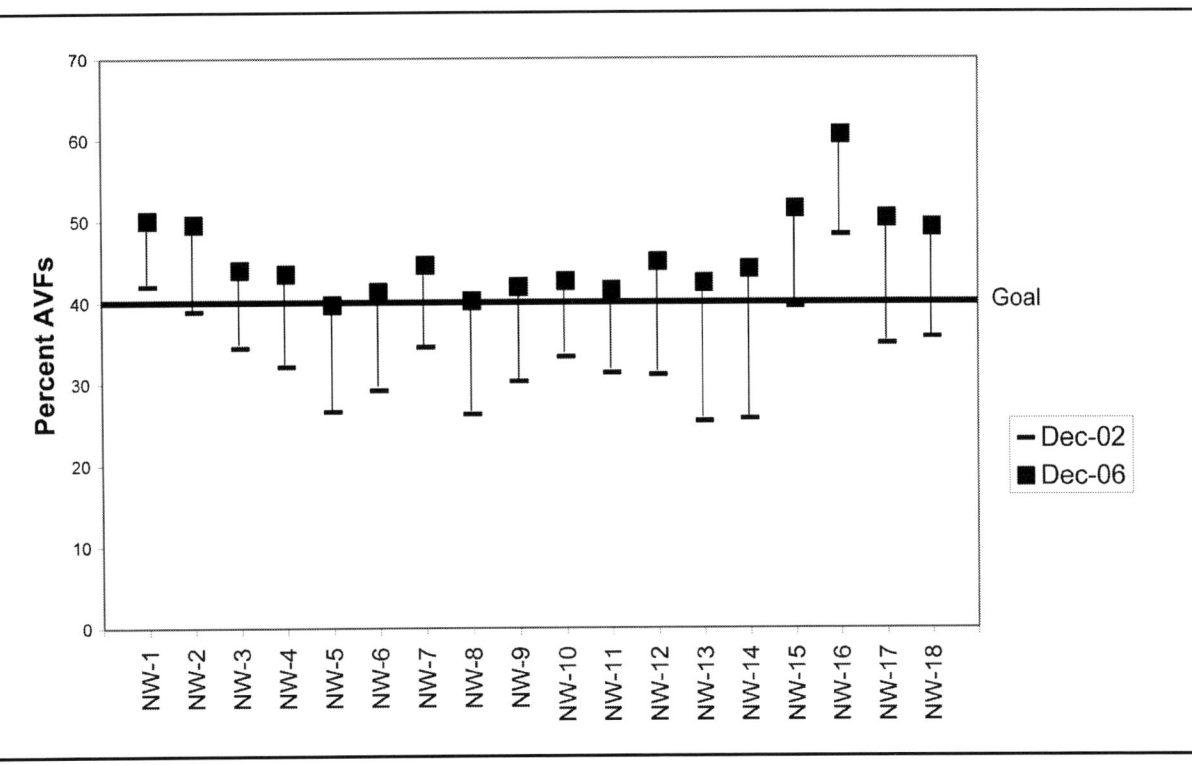

Every region of the United States attained substantial improvement in results, with all of the poorest performers in 2002 attaining or surpassing the national goal. Even the highest performers in 2002 continued to improve. Used with permission.

established relationships and communication channels with their local dialysis facilities and regional stakeholders. Their previous experience and training prepared them to learn and apply spread theory and strategies effectively.

Coordination of the Existing Structure Through a Clearly Defined Nodal Network

The Fistula First project was designed with a high level of coordination and communication among CMS, the ESRD networks, and regional stakeholders. The ability to share tools through a common extranet, to regularly convene for in-person meetings and teleconferences, and to have access to each others' expertise through a listserve enabled lessons to be shared and successes to be replicated and adapted quite rapidly. Maintaining the lines of communication and basic infrastructure throughout the project and focusing on aligning activities with strategies and goals also helped keep the system on track. Historically, health care organizations that become engaged in an improvement project want to "get going" with interventional activities immediately without doing adequate planning and set-up activities at the front end.

A Well-Known and Active Clinical Chair

Because communication through social and professional networks is so critical to the success of spread initiatives, it was extremely helpful to have a clinical chair who was not only recognized nationally for his work in this area but was willing to make himself available at numerous group events, as well as for individual conversations and correspondence.

Cooperation with CMS

There were three major areas in which CMS was able to strengthen the project.

- **Reimbursement.** Historically, a barrier to placing AVFs in larger numbers of patients has been the lack of reimbursement for "vessel mapping" procedures that allow physicians to study the patient's anatomy and identify the best options for placing an AVF. As the Fistula First initiative got underway and began to show success, a parallel effort at CMS resulted in a ruling and new government code to permit reimbursement for vessel mapping. By removing an important barrier, CMS signaled to the field that it was willing to align its policies with a national goal, thereby increasing the effort's credibility and providing "good news" that was amplified by the ESRD network staff in their outreach to clinicians. This accomplishment also established CMS as a critical partner and stakeholder in the project.

- **Assistance with Data Collection.** Prior to the Fistula First project, data on fistula prevalence were collected only once per year—too infrequently to be useful to the networks in assessing or revising their spread strategies. A team effort among CMS, the ESRD networks, and the large dialysis organizations resulted in a single data collection framework for the entire United States. This, for the first time, permitted data representing between 90% and 98% of all dialysis patients to be available on a monthly basis. Having frequent data allowed the team to see where significant improvements were occurring so that they could be studied and adapted by all the networks.

- **CMS Dedication of Resources.** CMS dedicated resources to this project not only through the ESRD network contracting process but also in support of the expanded Fistula First Breakthrough Initiative. Although the majority membership of the expanded project consists of volunteers, some budgetary allowances for part-time staff, meetings, conference phone lines, Web site support, and printing of educational materials has provided the initiative with the ability to tackle important issues that arise, as well as impetus for the ongoing spread of the project messages.

Identification of Clinician Champions

Finding expert, accomplished clinicians at the local level was a key strategy and helped drive the success of this initiative. These champions represented a range of expertise—surgeons, nephrologists, internists, nurses, technicians, interventionalists, and, in some cases, even dialysis patients. However, physicians with responsibility for patient referrals have been key, and vascular surgeons have taken on that leadership role in many regions of the United States. One of the lessons of this project has been the acknowledgement that early adopters are not necessarily the most successful facilities or practitioners. "Success" that can be translated into lessons for the community came from both the > 40% AVF facilities and the lower-level facilities willing to work hard and make improvements. Some of the early adopters who led significant improvement in initially low-AVF facilities presented excellent models for the late adopters, who tended to dismiss the high-AVF facilities as somehow "unique." The message from the low-AVF facilities, the proverbial "if-we-can-do-it-so-can-you," is difficult to ignore. Harnessing the energy of champions from all engaged facilities definitely contributed to the spread of this project.

Conclusion

The success of the Fistula First initiative is meaningful primarily in the lives of patients who have received AVFs who might otherwise have received types of vascular access that are less safe and effective. Gains in AVF use continue to accrue at unprecedented rates, with AVF prevalence of 45.4% through February 2007, the most recent data available. On the basis of the initiative's success, CMS announced on March 17, 2005, that the national goal for AVF use had been increased to 66%, an ambitious goal that the United States appears to be on track to meet. The human benefits of lower complications, fewer hospitalizations, and a vascular access that remains useful for a longer period of time are incalculable.

The national significance of the Fistula First initiative was recently highlighted in testimony before the House Committee on Ways and Means. Said Leslie Norwalk, acting administrator for CMS[14]:

> While all efforts under the ESRD Quality Initiative are significant, the Fistula First Breakthrough Initiative is particularly noteworthy. Under the initiative, facilities submit data to Medicare contractors charged with quality review of dialysis facilities ("ESRD Network Organizations") to facilitate a more coordinated approach to care. The initiative has led to a significant increase in the use of AV fistulas in treating dialysis patients—a measure associated with considerable reductions in avoidable hospitalization and death for ESRD beneficiaries.

The project has made a lasting impact on the work of the ESRD networks, which now have an effective and reusable set of skills for spreading other practices that may lead to better and more efficient patient care. Similarly, CMS has a blueprint that may be applied to other health care improvements in the future.

The analyses upon which this publication is based were performed under Contract Number 500-03-NW18, entitled "End-Stage Renal Disease Network Organization" for the region of Southern California, sponsored by the Centers for Medicare & Medicaid Services (CMS), Department of Health and Human Services (DHHS). The content of this publication does not necessarily reflect the views or policies of the DHHS, nor does mention of trade names, commercial products, or organizations imply endorsement by the U.S. government. The author assumes full responsibility for the accuracy and completeness of the ideas presented. This article is a direct result of the Health Care Quality Improvement Program initiated by CMS, which has encouraged identification of quality improvement projects derived from analysis of patterns of care, and therefore required no special funding on the part of this contractor. Ideas and contributions to the author concerning experience in engaging with issues presented are welcome.

The success of this project is due to the active support and participation of literally hundreds of project partners. The authors wish to acknowledge several who played an especially active role. From CMS: Stephen Jencks, M.D., M.P.H.; Brady Augustine, M.S.; Jefferson Rowland, M.Sc.; David Hunt, M.D.; Gina Clemons; and Judy Goldfarb. From the ESRD networks: Doug Marsh, executive director of Network 18 and the Network Coordinating Center; all the executive directors, quality improvement directors, and staff of the ESRD networks. The following individuals served as members of the expert panel or as members of the National Leadership Group: Anatole Besarab, M.D., Henry Ford Hospital; Deborah Brouwer, R.N., Allegheny General Hospital; Jeannette Cain, QI director, Network 9/10; Janet Crow, M.B.A., administrator, Forum of ESRD Networks; Leslie Dinwiddie, M.S.N., R.N., F.N.P., E.N.N., consultant; Richard Gray, M.D., Medstar Health; Maureen Herget, R.N., V.P., C.Q.M., Fresenius Medical Care; Toros Kapoian, M.D., UMDNJ – Robert Wood Johnson Medical School; Jennie Kitsen, executive director ESRD Network 1; Cathy Lewis, chair of the Patient and Family Council of the National Kidney Foundation; Donna Mapes, Dialysis Outcomes and Practice Patterns Study, Amgen, Inc.; Allen R. Nissenson, M.D., David Geffen School of Medicine at UCLA; Vo D. Nguyen, M.D., Renal Care Group of the Northwest; Michael Lazarus, M.D., senior vice president and medical director, Fresenius Medical Care; Darlene Rogers, executive director, Intermountain End-Stage Renal Disease Network, Inc.; John Sadler, president and CEO, Independent Dialysis Foundation; Barry M. Straube, M.D., Centers for Medicare & Medicaid Services; Marilyn Swartz, R.N., educator, National Kidney Foundation; Jack Work, M.D., Emory University; and Mike Zecca, ESRD patient. From the Institute for Healthcare Improvement: Kevin M. Nolan, M.A., improvement advisor; and Rebecca Steinfield, project manager.

References

1. Centers for Medicare & Medicaid Services: *Fistula First Breakthrough Initiative.* http://www.cms.hhs.gov/ESRDQualityImproveInit/04_FistulaFirstBreakthrough.asp#TopOfPage (accessed Jul. 11, 2007).
2. U.S. Renal Data System, 2006 Annual Data Report: *Atlas of End-State Renal Disease in the United States.* Bethesda, MD: National Institutes of Health, National Institute of Diabetes and Digestive and Kidney Diseases, 2006. http://www.usrds.org/adr.htm (accessed Jul. 11, 2007).
3. Hakim R., Himmelfarb J.: Hemodialysis access failure: A call to action. *Kidney Int* 54:1029–1040, Oct. 1998.
4. Bay W.H., Van Cleef S., Owens M.: The hemodialysis access: Preferences and concerns of patients, dialysis nurse and technicians, and physicians. *Am J Nephrol* 18(5):379–383, 1998.
5. Gibson K.D., et al.: Vascular access survival and incidence of revisions: A comparison of prosthetic grafts, simple autogenous fistulas, and venous transposition fistulas from the United States Renal Data System Dialysis Morbidity and Mortality Study. *J Vasc Surg* 34:694–700, Oct. 2001.
6. Rodriguez J.A., et al.: The function of permanent vascular access. *Neph Dial Transplant* 15:402–408, Mar. 2001.
7. Nassar G.M., Ayus J.C.: Infectious complications of the hemodialysis access. *Kidney Int* 60:1–13, Jul. 2001.
8. Eggers P.W., Milan R.: Trends in vascular access procedures and expenditures in Medicare's ESRD program. In Mitchell L.H. (ed.): *Vascular Access for Hemodialysis—VII.* Chicago: WL Gore & Precept Press, 2001, pp. 1–23.
9. U.S. Department of Health and Human Services: *Healthy People 2010: Understanding and Improving Health,* 2nd ed. Chapter 4: Chronic Kidney Disease. Washington, DC: U.S. Government Printing Office, Nov. 2000.
10. National Kidney Foundation (NKF): *NKF-DOQI Clinical Practice Guidelines for Vascular Access.* New York City: NKF, 1997.
11. *Fistula First Outcomes Dashboard.* http://www.esource.net/downloads/cds/fistulafirst/fistulafirstdashboard.pdf (accessed Jul. 13, 2007).
12. Greenwood R.N., et al.: Vascular access use in Europe and the United States: Results from the DOPPS. *Kidney Int* 61:305–316, Jan. 2002.
13. Nguyen V.D., Griffith C., Treat L.: A multidisciplinary approach to increasing AV fistula creation. *Nephrol News Issues* 17(7):54–56, 58, 60, 2003.
14. Statement of Leslie V. Norwalk, acting administrator, Centers for Medicare & Medicaid Services. Testimony before the House Committee on Ways and Means, Dec. 6, 2006.

Chapter 7
Insights and Conclusions

Kevin M. Nolan, M.A.
Marie W. Schall, M.A.

Spread can happen spontaneously. We believe, though, that developing, executing, and refining a plan for spread provides an opportunity to achieve desired outcomes in a specific time frame. The case studies in this book support this belief. We should not confuse planning for spread with *mandating* adoption of new ideas (or practices). In the spread initiatives described in the case studies, the leaders and spread teams did not mandate but rather facilitated the adoption of new ideas. At times, the facilitation took different courses but was guided by many of the same principles—which are included in the Framework for Spread (Chapter 1). The Framework for Spread allows flexibility for health care organizations to apply key spread principles to match their resources and existing structures.

In the case studies, organizations took different approaches to spread, as appropriate to the size and structure of the target populations. In large organizations such as Ascension Health, formal and informal groupings within the organization, such as regions or service lines, need to be leveraged. When the target population for spread is within a community, such as the National Vascular Access Improvement Initiative to spread fistula use for dialysis care (the Fistula First initiative), the natural structure within the community can be leveraged, but some entity—in this case, the Centers for Medicare & Medicaid Services (CMS)—is needed to provide leadership and gather resources. National, state, and local government agencies, professional associations, and Quality Improvement Organizations might serve this role.

As part of their spread plans, organizations undertook certain activities within the three connected phases of the framework: determining organizational readiness for spread, developing an initial spread plan, and executing and refining the spread plan. For example, all organizations deployed methods of communication to move adopters from awareness to decision and from decision to action. The communication activities varied, though, depending on existing communication channels and resources. We can learn from the similarities and differences in the spread activities in the case studies. Some of the activities are described in the sections that follow.

Organizational Readiness for Spread

Strategic Importance
To allow for sufficient support and resources for a spread initiative, senior leaders within an organization should connect the initiative with a key strategic objective. This was the case with the initiative to eliminate facility-acquired pressure ulcers at St. Vincent's Medical Center. As

this initiative spread throughout the Ascension Health system, the board of directors designated it as one of a small set of priorities. Leaders throughout Ascension Health then aligned incentives with performance in the prevention of pressure ulcers for all eligible associates. Because the prevention of pressure ulcers is primarily a nursing-driven process, the chief nursing officer (CNO) at St. Vincent's and, later, the CNOs throughout the system assumed executive sponsorship of the initiative.

At the New York City Health and Hospitals Corporation (HHC), the corporate goals, including the focus of the case study, improvement in chronic illness, were aligned with the goals set at each facility. Senior leaders (the chief executive officer and the senior vice presidents) attended and led sessions at the face-to-face meetings and recognized chronic disease improvement work throughout the organization. For example, nurse recognition awards were given to nursing leaders on chronic disease teams. Strategic alignment of goals was also evident at Beth Israel Medical Center in its efforts to spread the central line bundle. A spread initiative's strategic importance should be clear to all and not hidden within an overall objective of delivery of quality care. Fitting many different initiatives within this objective might lead many within the organization to question the priority of a given initiative.

The initiative to spread the set of safe handoff practices known as the Nurse Knowledge Exchange (NKE) at Kaiser Permanente (KP), although deemed an important undertaking, was not identified as a key strategic initiative. Leadership initially showed interest in the project because of their desire to create a clinical environment where nursing and other staff could thrive. However, once the pilot phase was completed, nurse executives did buy into implementation of the practice in hospitals across the system. Ultimately, senior leadership supported the need to standardize handoffs between nurses at change of shift and supported NKE as the vehicle with which to do it. This effort's success resulted from the development of the ideas at the frontline and the spread of the ideas through nursing peer networks. This might not have been possible if the process changes had required cooperation between multiple disciplines throughout the system. In such cases, leaders need to support and facilitate cooperation by making the spread initiative a strategic priority for the organization during the organizational readiness phase.

In a community setting, priorities can be established by an entity that will provide leadership for the spread initiative. This entity can then work with the key segments in the community to ensure that it is a priority for each segment. CMS, along with the End-Stage Renal Disease (ESRD) networks, played this role in the Fistula First initiative. CMS supported the formation of a spread team, whose members included representatives from CMS and the ESRD networks. The team developed partnerships with large dialysis organizations, professional organizations, and the National Kidney Foundation to support the effort. CMS also worked with the large dialysis organizations to develop a standard measurement system.

Role Definition

Although it is essential that senior leaders support the spread effort, they are usually not involved on a day-to-day basis. We have observed that successful spread initiatives, such as those represented in the case studies, dedicate resources to oversee and manage the spread effort. These resources will vary on the basis of the size of the target population and the scope of the ideas being spread. For the reduction of central line–associated bloodstream infections at Beth Israel, Dr. Brian Koll was the day-to-day manager and, as the chief of infection control, served as the sponsor. Dr. Koll provided sufficient resources to manage and support an initiative of this size and scope. HHC created a spread team that organized and supported the work of teams within their collaboratives, which were the HHC's main communication method. For larger spread initiatives, structured oversight teams, spread teams, and day-to-day managers with specific roles were identified. For example, to support the hospital teams' spread of NKE, KP created a national team and regional teams. The national team provided the national leadership, change package, coaching, project management, and measurement tracking. The regional teams provided specific leadership and support within each region. Day-to-day management and monitoring of the spread project for both the regional and national teams was the responsibility of the national project manager. Such levels of support were also developed for the

Fistula First initiative and the spread initiative at Ascension Health, and the case studies provide examples of the positions involved and their functions.

Successful Sites

In each of the case studies, members of the spread team developed and carried out a plan to document and build evidence for the new ideas. They first developed a collection of the ideas that were predicted to achieve the spread initiative's goals. In some cases, the evidence-based ideas were already fairly well documented. For example, HHC tested tools, protocols, and other resources about specific changes in care that were organized around the Chronic Care Model. Beth Israel used evidence-based practices collected as the central line bundle.

In situations where good ideas existed but were not well documented, such as for the Fistula First initiative, KP's NKE, and Ascension Health's initiative to eliminate facility-acquired pressure ulcers, the managers of the spread initiative convened a meeting where persons from within or outside an organization with knowledge about and success with the topic were brought together to share ideas. The result was a succinct package of ideas that sites in the target population could begin to test.

Once the initial ideas were gathered and packaged, the spread teams undertook activities to build evidence and refine the ideas by testing them in some units in the target population. In some of the case studies, criteria were used to select the initial sites. Ascension Health reviewed charts of patients who had developed pressure ulcers in the previous six months. The review revealed an increased risk for patients with one or more comorbidities among four diagnoses. The spread team shared this information with specific units, and the staff was eager to initiate the work. The spread team learned that illuminating the problem often facilitates the decision to adopt the changes. At KP, an assessment of readiness was conducted to identify units with the best chance of success. Beth Israel included units from its two hospitals. At HHC, each facility was asked to assemble a team to participate in its first collaborative.

The spread initiative experience in the case studies suggests two key points about successful sites:

1. Some of the spread teams used criteria to solicit participants. None of the sites, however, were forced to join the work.

2. The ideas that were spread were developed initially from the literature and from observation and experience of existing successful sites. The extent to which the ideas were documented varied. Each spread team, though, identified a few sites to test and implement the ideas. The successes in these initial sites built evidence for the ideas within the target population and were used in a communication plan to attract others to the work.

Developing and Executing the Spread Plan

If an organization or a community is ready for a spread initiative, it should develop an initial plan to guide its efforts. The first step in developing a plan is the documentation of an aim for spread. As an explicit statement documenting what an organization hopes to achieve in its spread initiative, the spread aim is the foundation of the plan. It also keeps the spread team focused and allows for communication of the intent of the spread initiative throughout the organization. Each organization in the case studies crafted a spread aim and then developed a spread plan to accomplish it.

An organization should include four components in its spread aim. For example, the four key components of Ascension Health's aim for spread were as follows:
- **The ideas being spread.** The principal ideas spread were head-to-toe skin assessments, risk assessments at every shift, and implementation of the SKIN bundle for patients at risk.
- **The target population.** All patients admitted to Ascension Health facilities
- **The time frame for the spread activities.** Full implementation at St. Vincent's Medical Center, the alpha site, by December 2005 and systemwide by 2007
- **The target levels of system performance.** Elimination of facility-acquired pressure ulcers throughout Ascension Health

For the case studies on improving dialysis care and safe handoff practices, the aim should have included a succinct statement of the ideas being spread. The inclusion of a specific time frame would have enhanced the aim statement for the case studies on the prevention of central line–associated bloodstream infections and for the redesign of chronic illness care (whose statement would also have benefited from specific numeric goals).

The spread plan outlines the methods an organization or a community intends to use to link those who have knowledge and experience with a new set of ideas and practices and the potential adopters of those ideas and practices. As stated in Chapter 1, the spread plan should address three areas: organizational structure, communication, and measurement and feedback.

Organizational Structure

Spread leaders should consider how closely and in what ways individuals within their organizations or communities are linked together through formal reporting or communication channels. KP created leadership teams at the national, regional, and facility levels to identify and develop pilot units, provide information and support, and measure progress and provide feedback to adopter units. It also built on an already existing labor management partnership structure to strengthen the initiative's position within the organization. Ascension Health used the nursing leadership structure at the national and facility levels to ensure that the necessary education and support were provided to frontline staff. Smaller organizations can also take advantage of formal relationships between pilot and adopter units. Spread leaders at Beth Israel were able to reach those involved in central line insertion through staff meetings in each of the intensive care units (ICUs) in its two-hospital system within a relatively short period.

In the Fistula First initiative, the existing structure of 18 End-Stage Renal Disease networks enabled the simultaneous initiation of the spread effort. Each network developed and executed a spread plan connected to the national effort. Structures were built, however, to connect the networks and, as with medical advisory boards, for example, to assist them in reaching the dialysis centers in their regions and the associated clinical specialists. When organizational structures among adopter sites do not exist, spread leaders can explore ways to create relationships and communication channels.

Organizational structures may also need to be enhanced as improvements developed in the pilot site are brought to full scale across an organization. For example, as the number of facilities and clinics in the HHC spread effort grew, the spread leaders recognized the need for an electronic decision-support system and an information technology infrastructure to enable pilot clinics to expand the number of patients reached by their interventions as well as to support the involvement of ever larger numbers of clinics. KP realized that the system's ability to bring the NKE system of practices to large numbers of units hinged on the practices' integration with the EHR that was also being implemented. A paper system, while effective as a temporary process, could not be implemented effectively and efficiently on a systemwide scale.

Communication

Developing and executing a communication plan is at the heart of any successful spread effort. An effective communication plan involves both identifying methods for attracting potential adopters and assisting them in taking action to adopt the changes.

A number of methods can be used to effectively build awareness. KP used an emotionally powerful video that recounted a case in which a child died as a result of errors reflecting handoff and other communication issues to motivate nurses to improve patient safety through improved communication at shift change. Ascension Health used comparative data from pilot and nonpilot units to persuade nurses that the elimination of facility-acquired pressure ulcers is an achievable goal. In addition, it held the systemwide Pressure Ulcer Summit to share the work of the pilot units and recruit additional facilities and units to the effort. Beth Israel used a series of presentations to all the ICUs in its two hospitals to raise awareness about central line infections and report comparative data from the pilot and nonpilot units. Data were also shared through newsletters, e-mail, posters in the units, and in-services. HHC encouraged the initial collaborative teams to present their work locally, such as at board committee meetings and external conferences. As the work progressed and more and more clinics became involved, participation became the norm, and it was more difficult for clinics to remain on the sidelines. The national leaders of the Fistula First initiative developed a set of standard communication resources such as videotapes and slide presentations that were targeted to key disciplines such as nephrologists and vascular access surgeons. At the regional level, project leaders used available communication channels, such as workshops, teleconferences, mailings, and online methods to reach their target audiences.

As adopters move from awareness about the existing problem and potential improvements to making the decision that they are ready to take action, they need information, support, guidance, and encouragement to implement the changes. Each organization should consider a number of factors, including the number of target units, its structure and culture, the nature of the interventions, and the available resources, in designing the communication system to support spread.

Ascension Health's communication plan for supporting adopters involved linking the work of St. Vincent's, as the alpha site, with the other 65 acute care hospitals in the system. Nursing units at hospitals that committed to the project following the Pressure Ulcer Summit participated in a national affinity group. The group was linked through monthly conference calls and a listserve that provided an opportunity for participants to share issues, raise questions, and obtain advice and guidance from St. Vincent's and a few additional hospitals that piloted the changes. At each hospital, the CNO and his or her leadership team decided whether to involve the nursing units on a unit-by-unit basis or in a housewide "go-live" process and provided the organizational leadership for the project.

Beth Israel also used a hospital-unit structure, in this case involving the ICUs, stepdown units, and emergency departments in its two hospitals. Following the initial pilot work at the three pilot ICUs, additional units were introduced to the central line bundle through in-services that were provided by the chief of infection control, the pilot units' physician and nursing champions, and, ultimately, other critical care unit staff. New units were brought into the spread effort on the basis of their response to information about the pilot units' work that was broadly shared through newsletters, e-mail, posters, department meetings, and grand rounds. The new units received data as feedback on their progress and support from the physician and nursing champions from the pilot units.

The key feature of KP's communication plan was the involvement of successive waves of nursing units in adopting the NKE process. At the hospital level, units were selected on the basis of interest and readiness. Once identified, the units were supported by a project lead at each facility. The project leads received coaching and support in their role as spread leaders through a collaborative structure involving an initial face-to-face meeting and regular conference calls, a listserve, and an extranet. Initially, because most of the participating hospitals did not have pilot units, the national team organized conference calls for all participating nursing units to share information about the elements of the NKE (as developed by the pilot units). However, as experience with NKE grew within each hospital, the project lead was able to coordinate sharing and support of the units through meetings and/or individual coaching.

HHC used a formal collaborative structure involving periodic in-person meetings of frontline teams and faculty, with conference calls, regular progress reports, and online resources to support action in local clinics. The spread eventually encompassed additional patients within the initial population of focus for the pilot teams, additional clinical conditions beyond the initial focus on diabetes and heart failure, and additional facilities. The expertise on how to improve chronic illness care was first provided by external consultants and a core of internal clinical leaders. As the collaborative grew, additional internal experts emerged, who provide coaching and support to newer teams. Site visits and meetings at clinics involving improvement staff, outside experts, and team members from other facilities were also used to foster sharing and accelerate adoption.

The national and network leaders of the Fistula First initiative developed a resource kit of tools, protocols, forms, and journal articles to facilitate adoption. To reach an audience with whom they had little influence or experience, the dialysis centers sponsored special informational sessions and provided material particularly for the vascular access surgeons to build awareness of and interest in the project, as well as technical information about the improvements. Dr. Spergel, a nationally recognized vascular access surgeon, played a key role in reaching the surgeons. At the regional level, some large dialysis organizations set up their own training programs for vascular access staff, while other centers trained groups of clinical "coaches" who were willing to serve as mentors to their peers. In other areas, groups of "vascular access clubs" began self-organization to offer mutual support.

Mentors were also used in the other case study examples, including KP, which identified "super users" from the initial wave of the collaborative to serve as internal coaches and advisers to subsequent units. In a large spread effort, an organization's communication plan should entail the recruitment and development of such mentors in each facility and/or region so as not to overburden one or two mentors. Recruiting additional mentors also enables organizations to involve them in more one-on-one peer coaching. For example, Ascension Health used bedside teaching as a way to enhance nurses' knowledge about the prevention of pressure ulcers.

Once a communication plan is under way, it becomes the responsibility of the spread leaders to listen to the adopters to learn how to strengthen the plan and enhance information and support for the adopters. Beth Israel used a formal root cause analysis (RCA) process to review each occurrence of a central line infection to identify issues that might hinder wider adoption of the advocated idea or practice. One RCA empowered nurses to confront physicians who are not following the standard protocols. At KP, spread leaders learned of nurses' frequent reluctance to conduct bedside rounds because of concerns about a possible violation of sharing information that they had previously shared only in private with their peers. This led to the development of scripts that nurses could practice and then use at the bedside. Storytelling by nurses as part of the process of sharing their experience with the NKE practice helped to draw more nurses into the spread effort.

Listening to adopters can also identify infrastructure or transition issues that, if not addressed, might impede widespread adoption of the ideas being spread. Preexisting regulations can sometimes be a real or perceived barrier. KP was able to address the issue of a perceived violation of the Health Insurance Portability and Accountability Act by reassuring nurses who were concerned about bedside rounds, as described. At Beth Israel, an RCA led to the development of a central line cart with standard equipment so that staff would be able to more easily follow the recommended protocol.

Measurement and Feedback

During a spread initiative, two different types of measures are useful: (1) outcome measures that demonstrate the impact on system performance and (2) measures that demonstrate the extent of the spread of the new ideas. The outcome measures should reflect the aggregate level of performance of the target population. For the initiative to eliminate facility-acquired pressure ulcers at Ascension Health, data were initially monitored for St. Vincent's Medical Center, the alpha site. As the ideas were spread, data were aggregated and displayed for hospitals throughout the system. A similar measurement approach was used for central line–associated bloodstream infections at Beth Israel. HHC developed a registry to track clinical outcomes to assess system performance. For the Fistula First initiative, a data collection system was developed in cooperation between CMS and the large dialysis organizations to make available national data on the rate of fistula use. This data collection system could also display the data by network (that is, by region of the United States). Data on fistula use were also available by dialysis facility. KP established four outcome measures: falls with injury, patient satisfaction, staff satisfaction, and reduction in incidental overtime. KP had preliminary data from the pilot sites indicating improvement in patient and staff satisfaction and from one medical center showing a reduction in overtime. KP is now in the process of collecting outcome data for each unit that has fully implemented NKE. This is an important activity because it enables KP to provide feedback to adopters and refine its spread plan accordingly.

Spread teams, which use data on the rate of spread to monitor the extent of the adoption of the ideas in the target population, will often find that collecting and displaying such data is not easy. The Fistula First initiative case study acknowledged the important limitation of a lack of information on the extent of adoption of the ideas. However, each dialysis facility's access to its data on its own fistula use enabled the day-to-day managers to identify the units where adoption was lagging and consequently were in need of coaching.

The case studies from Ascension Health and KP each described the collection of data on the rate of spread but did not include the resulting summary data. Beth Israel reported that compliance with the central line bundle took about 60 days but provided data (which confirmed this finding) for only one ICU. The case study from HHC provided graphs showing the number of patients in the chronic disease registry and the number of physicians involved in the improvement work, but graphs on the actual rate of adoption of the ideas in the target population would have been an enhancement.

It is critical that spread teams track the rate of adoption. Even in the absence of efforts to track rate of spread for the entire target population, spread teams can still gather information on the extent of spread from reports or verbal contact from a sample of organizations. Information on the adoption of ideas, linked with data on outcomes, provides the foundation for a spread team's development and maintenance of a feedback system for adopters. A spread team should provide for support of organizations, including assistance with communication, technical support, and measurement, when needed.

Another important feedback loop is the one that captures the growing knowledge base as more and more sites adapt the ideas to their local situations. The Fistula First initiative developed a Web site to collect tools and resources to support the spread efforts. HHC posted specific changes in care and tools that emerged from successful teams on an intranet site dedicated to the chronic disease improvement work. At Beth Israel, RCAs were conducted within 24 hours of each central line bloodstream infection to develop and document knowledge to improve the effectiveness of the central line bundle.

Maintaining the Gains

A number of the case studies in this book spoke to the factors that have contributed to their ability to sustain the improvements realized through their spread efforts. Common themes include continued data collection and sharing of results at the leadership and unit levels, leadership attention and involvement, the use of protocols and standard procedures and ongoing training to support their use, and the central role of unit managers in continuing responsibility for and oversight of the new system.

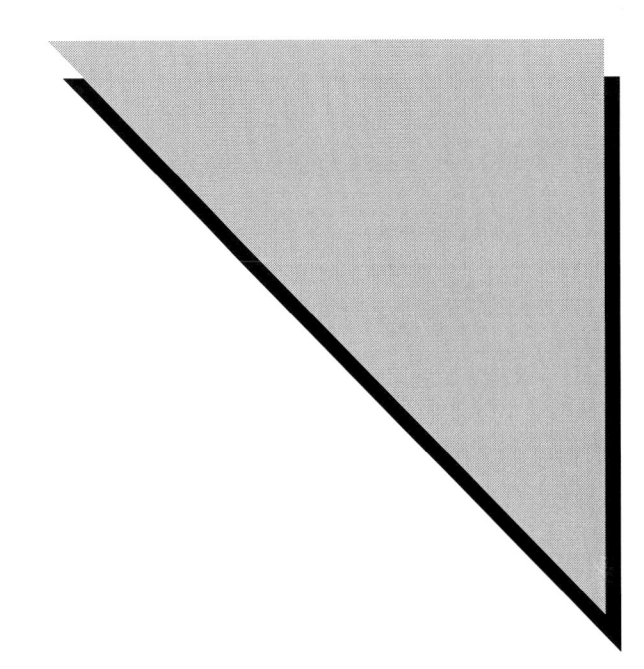

Index

A

Access to health care
    Framework for spread and, 2
    improving, 5
    strategic planning for, 3
Adopters
    communication issues, 14, 117
    feedback issues, 15
    of Fistula First initiative, 110
    identification of, 16–17
    knowledge transfer by, 17, 19–20
    listening to, 118
    role of, 19
Adoption
    of change ideas, 101
    of Fistula First initiative, 101
    identifying barriers to, 16
    of new ideas, 6
    of NKE Collaborative, 70, 74
    rate of, 18, 74
    of SKIN bundle, 20, 30
    spread of ideas and, 12
Adverse drug events, 15
Aim statement
    components of, 10, 115
    examples of, 11
    for spread initiative, 10–11
Alpha site initiative
    cultural modification for, 27–28
    St. Vincent's Medical Center, 26–27, 36–37
Ambulatory care services, 78
Appointments. *See* Future appointments

Arteriovenous fistula (AVF)
    ESRD network goals and, 97, 102
    influencing use of, 98
    prevalence by network, 96
    purpose of, 95
    rate of, 96–97, 103, 108–110
Ascension Health system. *See also* Pressure ulcer elimination/prevention
    background, 25–26
    CNO group of, 34–36
    communication plan for, 116, 117, 118
    e-learning initiative by, 36–37
    insights and conclusions, 113
    priorities for action for, 26

B

Backlog
    defined, 8
    measurement of, 8–9
Beth Israel Medical Center
    background, 41–43
    central line bundle implementation at, 43–53
    communication plan for, 116, 117
    organizational readiness and, 114
Better ideas component, 1
Braden Scale for Predicting Pressure Sore Risk, 27, 29, 30
Breakthrough Series College, 71, 74
Breakthrough Series collaborative, 78, 83
Brooklyn hospital
    central line bundle implementation at, 44, 49
    reduction in CLABs at, 50

C

Caring Model, 58
Case studies
    Ascension Health system, 25–39
    Beth Israel Medical Center, 41–53
    Kaiser Permanente, 55–56
    National Vascular Access Improvement Initiative (Fistula First), 95–100
    New York City Health and Hospitals Corporation (HHC), 77–80
Centers for Disease Control (CDC), 107
Centers for Medicare & Medicaid Services (CMS), 95, 105, 106, 110–111
Central line-associated bloodstream infections (CLABs)
    central line bundle and, 42
    data collection of, 47, 48
    duration of days without, 52
    elimination of, 43
    incidence of, 41
    monitoring tool, 48
    mortality of, 42
    per 1,000 line days, 49
    principles, 44
    RCAs for, 45, 47
    reduction in, 50, 51
Central line bundle initiative
    benefits of, 52
    CLABs and, 42
    components of, 43
    implementation of, 43–45, 47, 50
    lessons learned from, 50, 53
    rate of compliance, 50
    role definition for, 114–115
    as spread initiative, 43
    spread of, 47, 50
    teams for, 44
    time line for, 49
Central-line insertion kit, 44, 46, 47
Central-line insertion technique, 45
Central venous catheters, 41, 96
Change package, 70–71
Chronic Care Model
    adapting disease management principles from, 78
    as a framework, 80
    HHC version of, 83, 86, 115

Chronic disease collaborative
    communication plan for, 83, 85–86, 89
    diabetes, 84, 90
    expansion of, 89–90
    goals and targets, 79, 80
    heart failure, 85
    intranet for, 80, 83, 86, 89
    leadership's role in, 78, 82–83
    lessons learned from, 92–93
    results of, 89–92
    specific ideas for, 83
    spread plan for, 80, 82, 89
    teams' role in, 78–80
    training for, 85–86
Chronic Illness Care program, 78
Chronic kidney disease (CKD), 105
Clinical information systems. *See* Information technology
Communication issues/plan
    for chronic disease collaborative, 83, 85–86, 89
    development of, 13–14, 23
    for Fistula First initiative, 103–104, 107–109, 117–118
    for NKE Collaborative, 62, 117–118
    nurse shift change and, 56
    for pressure ulcer elimination, 38, 116, 118
Communication of awareness
    spread plan and, 16–17
    worksheet for, 19
Community resources
    for diabetes management, 84
    HHC Care Model, 86

D

"Dashboard" data, 107, 108
Data collection
    of AVF rate, 107
    chronic disease collaborative and, 89
    of CLABs, 47
    Fistula First initiative, 99, 110, 118
    measurement and feedback and, 119
    of NKE Collaborative, 60, 65–67
Day-to-day manager
    activities for, 7
    for spread initiative, 4
    spread team for, 4

Decision support
    for diabetes management, 84
    for heart failure, 85
    HHC Care Model, 86
Delivery systems design
    for diabetes management, 84
    for heart failure, 85
    HHC Care Model, 86
Depression screening, 92
Diabetes management
    key changes for, 84
    tool kit, 87
Diabetes team, 79, 90
Dialysis centers
    data collection by, 110
    Fistula First initiative and, 103, 104
    reporting of AVF rate data by, 107
Dialysis therapy, defined, 95
Dietitians, 28

E

Education and training
    for chronic disease collaborative, 85–86
    for Fistula First initiative, 103, 106
    for NKE Collaborative, 65
    for pressure ulcer prevention, 29–30
Electronic health record (EHR)-KP HealthConnect, 56, 58
End-Stage Renal Disease (ESRD) networks
    communication issues, 103–104
    description of, 95
    Fistula First initiative's impact on, 111
    goals of, 97
    methods used to spread initiative, 104
    organizational readiness and, 114
    organizational structure and, 116
    spread activities, 102–103
    teams for, 99
Executive sponsor
    for NKE Collaborative, 62, 64
    role of, 4
    spread team for, 4

F

Facility-acquired pressure ulcers. *See* Pressure ulcers
Fistula First Breakthrough initiative, 100, 106, 110
Fistula First initiative
    adoption of, 101
    aim for, 95–98
    background, 95
    change ideas, 97, 99, 100
    communication plan for, 103–104, 107, 117–118
    conclusion about, 110–111
    Coordination Group for, 99, 103
    elements of, 98–99
    feedback system, 104–105
    implementation structure, 99–100
    important factors for success of, 108–110
    knowledge management system, 105
    leadership's role in, 99
    lessons learned from, 108–110
    measurement and feedback for, 118–119
    organizational structure and, 116
    quality measurement, 107
    results of, 108–109
    spread activities level for, 102–103
    spread plan for, 101–106
    teams for, 99
Framework for Spread
    components of, 1–2
    improving performance with, 2–3
    introduction to, 1
    phases of, 3
Future appointments, 9

H

Hand hygiene compliance, 45
Health care organization
    for diabetes management, 84
    for heart failure, 85
    HHC Care Model, 86
Health Insurance Portability and Accountability Act (HIPAA), 66, 118
Heart failure management
    key changes for, 85
    tool kit, 88
Heart failure team, 79, 91–92

Hemodialysis, 95, 96
HHC. *See* New York City Health and Hospitals Corporation (HHC)
Hospital Consumer Assessment of Healthcare Providers and Systems (H-CAHPS), 60
Hospital system
    barriers and methods and, 73–74
    social systems and networks in, 71
Hospital team
    for NKE Collaborative, 62
    support for, 65

I

Implementation Working Group, 105
Improvement infrastructure, xii
Information technology
    chronic disease collaborative and, 82
    for diabetes management, 84
    Fistula First initiative and, 105
    for heart failure management, 85
    HHC Care Model, 86
Institute for Healthcare Improvement (IHI), 27, 55, 71
Institute for Healthcare Improvement's 5 Million Lives Campaign, xii
Intranet for chronic disease collaborative, 80, 83, 86, 89
Iowa Health System
    displaying spread of ideas at, 17
    monitoring adverse drug events at, 14, 15
    tracking spread of ideas in, 16
iSBAR tool, 57, 60

K

Kaiser Permanente
    background, 55–56
    communication issues, 117
    NKE initiative aim for, 59–60
    organizational readiness and, 114
Knowledge management component, 2, 105
Knowledge transfer, 17, 19–20
KP Model of Care, 58

L

Labor Management Partnership (LMP), 73
Leadership
    for central line bundle, 43–44
    for chronic disease collaborative, 78, 80, 82, 83
    for Fistula First initiative, 99, 102, 103
    Framework for Spread and, 1
    NKE Collaborative and, 62, 65, 69, 71
    organizational readiness and, 114
    organizational structure and, 6, 8, 116
    for pressure ulcer elimination, 27, 28, 30, 35, 37
    for spread initiative, 3, 12

M

MacColl Institute for Healthcare Innovation, 78
Manhattan hospital
    central line bundle implementation at, 44
    rate of CLABs at, 49
Materials management, 47, 53
Measurement and feedback component, 2, 118–119
Measurement plan, 14–15, 24
Medication system, patient safety and, 11
Middle managers, role of, 20
Multiple sites
    linking of, 10
    taking advantage of, 12

N

National Healthcare Safety Network (NHSN), 44, 47, 49, 50
National Kidney Foundation, 114
National Pressure Ulcer Advisory Panel, 25, 29
National team, 62, 64
National Vascular Access Improvement Initiative. *See also* Fistula First initiative
    background, 95
    rationale and aim for spread, 95–98
New ideas
    adoption of, 6
    description of, 8–9
    importance of, 6
New York City Health and Hospitals Corporation (HHC)
    background, 77–78
    communication issues, 116, 117
    key changes by, 83–86, 89
    organizational readiness and, 114
    spread strategy, 81
NKE Collaborative. *See* Nurse Knowledge Exchange (NKE) Collaborative
Nurse shift change

NKE's impact on, 57–58
problem of, 56
template for, 57–59
Nurse Knowledge Exchange (NKE) Collaborative
  assessment phase of, 56
  changes in, 67, 69
  communication plan for, 117–118
  components of, 57–58
  conclusion about, 73, 75
  data collection and tools for, 65–67
  development of, 56–57
  discussion about, 69–74
  evolution of, 55
  formation of, 61–62
  as high-tech, 58–59
  implementation of, 64–65, 69, 70
  improvements with, 58
  innovation method for, 56–57
  lessons learned from, 73
  local and national, 72–73
  measurement and feedback for, 118–119
  model for spread and sustainability, 73
  organizational readiness and, 114
  organizational structure and, 116
  plan to spread, 60–69
  process measure questions related to, 66–68
  resources for, 63
  results of, 69
  role definition for, 114–115
  structure for spread, 72
  three-tier structure for, 62
  three-wave, 62, 64–65
  tools for success of, 72
Nursing leadership/staff
  central line bundle and, 45, 48
  NKE Collaborative and, 66, 69
  pressure ulcer elimination and, 28, 37

O

Opinion leaders, considerations for using, 14
Organizational readiness
  sample form, 22
  for spread initiative, 3–4
  strategic importance for, 113–114
Organizational structure
  communication plan and, 14
  considering changes in, 6, 8
  ESRD network and, 116
  Fistula First initiative and, 108–109
  for spread plan, 10, 12–13, 116
Organizations
  formal groupings in, 12
  infrastructure, 99

P

Partnerships with entities, 13
Patient-Health Questionnaire, 92
Patient safety
  effective medication system and, 11
  improving, 5
Physician offices and clinics, 5
Pilot sites
  communication issues, 116, 117
  measurement and feedback and, 118
  for NKE initiative, 56, 59, 60, 71
  nurse shift change and, 59, 61
  organizational structure and, 116
  for SKIN bundle, 28
Plan-do-study-act methodology, 44–45, 47
Pressure ulcer elimination/prevention
  discussion about, 37–39
  education plan for, 29–30
  key elements of, 36
  measurement and feedback for, 118–119
  monitoring of, 36
  results of, 33–34
  as spread initiative, 26
  spread of, 33–37
  support for, 35–36
  time line, 27
Pressure ulcers
  defined, 25
  downward trend of, 33–34
  incidence of, 25
  zero facility-acquired, 26, 33, 36, 39
Pressure Ulcer Summit, 34–35
Process measure questions
  NKE Collaborative, 66
  tracking of, 67–68
Project leads, 70–74
Project management
  leadership and, 71

NKE Collaborative, 65–67

Q

Quality improvement (QI) directors, 82, 99, 100, 108
Quality improvement (QI) initiative, 82, 95, 100
Quality improvement (QI) staff, 80, 82, 99, 102, 108
Quality Improvement Organizations, 105, 106

R

Regional team, 62, 64
Root cause analyses (RCAs)
 for CLABs, 45, 47, 118
 importance of, 47

S

Self management support
 for diabetes management, 84
 for heart failure, 85, 91
 HHC Care Model, 86
Set-up component, 1
Sites. See Multiple sites; Successful sites
SKIN bundle
 barriers to using, 39
 compliance tool, 32
 description of, 27
 implementation of, 30, 33–35
 monitoring of, 30, 33
 pilot units for, 28
 spread of, 33–37
Skin care, 29
Skin initiative poster, 30, 35
SKIN operations meetings, 28, 30, 33, 37
SKIN RISK alert reminder, 31
Social network/system
 chronic disease collaborative and, 82, 92
 Fistula First initiative and, 104
 of Framework for Spread, 2
 in hospital system, 71
Spread improvements, xi–xiii
Spread initiative
 aim statement for, 10–11
 central line bundle as, 43
 chronic disease collaborative as, 80
 day-to-day manager for, 4
 executive sponsorship for, 4

Fistula First initiative as, 95–108
 gathering ideas for, 4–6
 maintaining the gains for, 119
 measurement and feedback for, 118–119
 NKE Collaborative as, 59–69
 pressure ulcer elimination as, 26
 readiness for, 3–4, 22, 113–115
 review of, 19–20
 spread team for, 4
 use of incentives for, 6
Spread of ideas
 assessing, 7
 attributes for influencing, 5–6
 displaying, 17
 rate of, 18
 tracking, 16
Spread plan
 communication plan for, 13–14
 completeness and coverage of, 12–13
 development of, 23, 115–119
 executing and refining, 15–20, 22–24, 115–119
 feedback issues, 20
 for Fistula First initiative, 101–105
 measurement plan for, 14–15
 organizational structure for, 10, 12–13, 116
 time line, 22–24
Spread team
 for chronic disease collaborative, 78–80, 82
 communication plan by, 13–14
 description of ideas by, 8
 examples of, 5
 opinion leaders and, 14
 organizational structure and, 10
 for pressure ulcer elimination, 27
 role of, 10
 for spread initiative, 4
 spread plan execution by, 15–20
 worksheet for, 7
St. Vincent's Medical Center. See also Pressure ulcer elimination/prevention
 alpha site initiative, 26–27, 36–37
 introduction to, 25
 organizational readiness and, 113–114
 pilot units at, 28–29, 38–39
Strategic planning, 3–4, 10

Successful sites
    Brooklyn hospital, 44
    communicating work of, 6
    defined, 5
    description of ideas from, 6, 8
    Manhattan Hospital, 44
    replicating best practices from, 14, 115
    using representatives of, 12
Synthetic arteriovenous grafts, 96
System performance
    effective medication system and, 11
    measurement plan and, 14
    patient care and, 11

T

Target audiences
    activities undertaken by, 106
    chronic disease collaborative and, 83
    Fistula First initiative, 100, 103, 104, 107
    SKIN bundle, 34
Target population
    for chronic disease collaborative, 80
    communication issues, 13
    for Fistula First initiative, 113
    listening to, 15
    measurement plan for, 14
    monitoring of, 16–17
    SKIN bundle and, 26
    spread plan and, 6, 10
    successful sites and, 12
    time frame for spread and, 11

Target sites, 14
Time line
    central line bundle, 49
    pressure ulcer prevention, 27
    spread plan, 22–24
Tipping point, 16
Toolkits, Web-based, 83
Training. *See* Education and training
2004 Hill-Room International Pressure Ulcer Prevalence Survey, 28
2006 International Pressure Ulcer Prevalence Study, 25

U

Urgent Care Clinic, 9

V

Value-added care, 11
Vascular access, ways to achieve, 95–96
"Vessel mapping" procedures, 110
Veterans Health Administration (VHA)
    Framework for Spread and, 2–3
    ideas description by, 8–9
Veterans Integrated Service Networks (VISNs), 2

W

Web-based tool kits, 83
Wound Ostomy and Continence Nurses Society (WOCN), 25